THE ANTI INFLAMMATORY DIET

6 SIMPLE STEPS TO LIVING DISEASE FREE

DALE PINNOCK

CONTENTS

INTRODUCTION

Out of all of the conditions and health issues that I see in my clinic, almost all of them have an inflammatory component to them. It is such a key part of disease process and disease progression that it always ends up being some part of the picture, no matter what we are dealing with. Virtually every nutritional plan or supplement protocol that I come up with for my patients will have an inflammatory management element to them. There is a good reason for that. Inflammation drives disease. Period. Well, more specifically, a certain type of inflammation that can easily get out of control drives disease and managing it is vital.

Management of inflammation in the body has two benefits to it. Firstly, it will absolutely help to manage symptoms. If you have a condition like arthritis for example, you will be acutely aware of the impact that inflammation has on your daily life. That pain and swelling and joint dysfunction. That is inflammation in action. You will know what a difference managing and reducing this will make to your life. These types of conditions are the more obvious manifestations of inflammation.

But, did you know that inflammation, of a less obvious kind is actually the primary driver of all of the degenerative diseases that seem to plague us in later years. Those things that we just associate with ageing. The things that either fill our hospital wards or our GP surgeries. Inflammation is at the core of these. Think heart disease, type 2 diabetes, many cancers, even some mental health issues.

Managing this type of inflammation is one of the keys to long term good health and the reduction in our risk of degenerative disease, and our ability to recover. I have mentioned it in many of my previous books and in almost every interview I do we end up discussing chronic low grade inflammation. Understanding it and learning how to manage it is absolutely vital. That is why I decided to dedicate a whole book to the subject.

This book is for you if you have any inflammatory issues such as arthritis, eczema, acne, autoimmune conditions and well established inflammatory conditions. The plan in this book will provide relief and effective management of those issues rapidly and effectively. However, this book is also for you if you have any kind of metabolic disease. High blood pressure, high cholesterol, heart disease, type 2 diabetes and even mental health issues like depression. Or indeed you have a family history of such conditions and want to keep them at bay. Inflammation is the fan to their flame and calming it will send these conditions packing.

What Exactly Is Inflammation?

So what is it? Inflammation is a normal and necessary process in our body and it isn't all bad. It is a key protective mechanism that is vital to our very survival; a built-in response that helps us heal from the daily wear and tear of life, fight infections and repair damaged tissues efficiently. Without it we wouldn't last long at all. However, it also can have a less beneficial side. A side that can run ragged and cause chaos. When it runs unchecked or deviates from its intended purpose, it can start to damage our health in some very serious ways, as you will soon see.

To appreciate the value of inflammation, we need to look at its original purpose. In the simplest sense, it is how the body organises a defence against anything that might cause harm, be that a cut on your finger or an invading pathogen. Inflammation is a highly orchestrated process that ensures damaged tissues can mend properly, and that also allows the rapid transport of key immune cells to the site of infection or damaged tissue so they can get on with their job faster. Like so many biological systems, it needs to be activated appropriately and then deactivated once the threat has passed or the damaged tissue is on its way to healing. Problems can arise, however, when this well-regulated process gets stuck in a 'switched on' position. The innate healing force that is meant to protect can start to erode and disrupt normal function.

The best way to look at inflammation's significance is to see it as having two faces. One is very beneficial. Vital in fact. The other, we need to get to grips with and the one that causes all of the damage and chaos.

Let's start with the beneficial side of the picture. On one hand, there is the acute, short-lived inflammation that flares up in response to clear and present dangers like infection or injury. This variety is easy to recognise: think swollen ankles after a sprain, redness around a small wound, or the low-grade fever that signals your body is fighting a cold. These symptoms may be uncomfortable, but they are often short-lived and intended to help you recover. Once the healing is complete, the body stands down from its high alert, and you return to your usual state.

On the other hand, there is chronic, long-term, inflammation, which can persist without any obvious signs to the naked eye. It is what we refer to as sub clinical. You might go about your daily business not realising that, inside, your body has launched a simmering, persistent inflammatory response. Over time, this can show itself in a variety of ways, from nagging aches and daytime fatigue to a more general sense of feeling 'off'. In most cases though, it remains undetected until a more serious health issue arises. This is the covert aspect of inflammation, the one that lurks beneath the surface and has become a focus of cutting-edge health and medical research. This is going to be our focus and this is the type of inflammation that we can tackle with diet. This is the one we need to fight at all costs.

Few systems in the human body have such a wide range of effects. Inflammation, by its nature, touches on nearly every aspect of our physiology, in every part of our body. When it works as it should, we don't often notice it, except perhaps for the brief intervals when we experience a minor cut or bruise. When it misfires or overstays its welcome, the impact can be significant and catastrophic. Modern science has connected chronic, low-grade sub clinical inflammation to a range of common diseases and conditions, changing our understanding of what drives long-term health and vitality.

But why should we worry about inflammation at all, especially if most of us encounter it merely as a bit of soreness here and there? The reason is that inflammation can quietly accumulate over time if left unaddressed. Even in the absence of an obvious damaging event—like a sudden injury—small aggravations can add up, compounding daily micro-stresses into larger health concerns. Think of it as a drip, drip, drip effect, rather than a bursting pipe. Both situations can cause damage, but the steady leak is often more difficult to spot and, in many ways, more challenging to repair once it's done enough harm. That's the same deal here. Just because we do not have any obvious symptoms

A 21st-Century Challenge

It's often said that we live in an age of abundance. I suppose in a lot of ways that is true. But our quest for instant gratification and convenience has come back to bite us. Food is readily available—often too readily—and technological advances mean we move around less than at any point in human history. Meanwhile, the pace of life continues to accelerate, with many people juggling hectic work schedules and family commitments, leaving little time for rest or even a shred of self-care. This mix of factors plays havoc with our inflammatory systems, keeping them engaged far longer than nature intended.

In many ways, inflammation is a mirror reflecting our shift away from more balanced lifestyles. Our ancestors required acute inflammatory responses to survive the environmental threats of their day. They relied on quick bursts of energy for hunting or fighting, followed by regular periods of rest and nutrient-rich diets that were, of course, free from modern processing. By contrast, our current lifestyles are a potent mix of convenience foods, chronic stress, and minimal downtime, combining to disrupt the body's finely tuned systems. Modern life is mayhem. But, that does not mean we are hopeless and cannot improve things.

It's not all doom and gloom. By understanding what inflammation truly is—and how it can be leveraged or reined in—we can learn to read our bodies' signals more accurately and respond accordingly. Small changes in daily habits can deliver large benefits.

While the notion of an 'anti-inflammatory diet' may sound like a bit of a buzzword, there is avast amount to it. At its heart, it's about aligning our food and lifestyle choices with the body's inherent design, and respecting the natural processes that have evolved over millennia. By choosing more nutrient-dense foods, moving our bodies appropriately, and carving out time for recovery and rest, we essentially help the inflammatory system return to its core function: healing us swiftly when needed, then standing down.

It's crucial to recognise that inflammation doesn't exist in a vacuum. There's a close interrelationship between inflammation and other systems, including hormonal regulation, brain function, and metabolic health. The chapters that follow will illuminate these connections, but for now, know that inflammation goes hand in hand with understanding your overall well-being. When you learn what truly nourishes your body, you're often learning how best to maintain a healthy inflammatory response too.

How This Book Will Help

Rather than overwhelming you with too much scientific jargon, we'll progress step by step, covering the crucial points of inflammation's role in health. You'll learn where inflammation fits into your body's grand scheme, how it can shift from something good to something harmful, and the most up-to-date evidence on how dietary patterns and certain lifestyle choices can tame or intensify those inflammatory processes. Along the way, we'll touch upon straightforward, practical methods you can adopt to tip the scales in favour of a balanced inflammatory response.

As you move through the chapters, you'll see how inflammation underpins a great deal of what we experience physically and even mentally. You'll also have the chance to explore how small tweaks can have a huge effect on your day-to-day well-being. Whether your goal is to manage a known health condition or simply to age gracefully and protect yourself from degenerative disease, comprehending inflammation can be a major step forward.

Ultimately, this journey is about reclaiming a sense of control over your own health. Rather than viewing inflammation as an ominous, uncontrollable force, you'll come to see it as part of a vital, adaptive system that you can influence. We'll delve deeper into the complexities of this system and, crucially, unravel how an anti-inflammatory approach can support everything from immune resilience to joint function, cognitive performance, and more.

Above all, think of this exploration as an opportunity: an opportunity to reframe what it means to 'eat well', to discover the dynamic relationship between food, body, and mind, and to unlock a toolkit of strategies that can help you thrive. By the end of this book, you should feel both informed and empowered, ready to integrate the anti-inflammatory diet and lifestyle insights into your everyday life in a manner that feels sustainable, personalised, and entirely your own.

The Diet-Inflammation Connection

When we look at how our diet has changed over the decades, it is a wonder we are even standing. Many of the things that we consume are as far away from food as we could possibly get and certainly do not resemble the kinds of foods our bodies were designed to eat in order to thrive. Our body is that good at surviving that it pushes through. But the consequences are significant. Amongst all the lifestyle factors that influence our inflammatory state—sleep, stress, movement—diet stands out as one of the most potent. After all, we have to eat each day; the question is, what are we choosing to eat, and how does that shape our internal environment? Too many of us overlook the impact that diet has on physiology. But, when you think about it, the food that we eat and the nutrients and chemicals it provides influence virtually every single aspect of our physiology, either positively or negatively.

Historically, our ancestors relied on real, unprocessed foods. Of course they did. There wasn't a fast food joint or manufacturing plant around was there? They ate what they could hunt, forage, or cultivate, and the human body evolved within that framework. As far as our body is concerned, we still live in the same conditions. Our physiology has not evolved as rapidly as our outside World. In those ancient conditions, acute inflammation served its intended purpose: to mend wounds quickly and fend off infections or parasites. Chronic inflammation would have been a less common phenomenon, partly because people were not routinely exposed to high amounts of highly processed, calorie-rich, nutrient-poor foods.

Fast-forward to our modern era, where many of us have access to an abundance of convenient, heavily processed items that have little resemblance to the raw ingredients from which they originated. We consume these foods at a frequency our ancestors would find remarkable, often without fully understanding the impact on our immune and metabolic systems. Over time, research has revealed that diets high in refined sugars, artificial additives, and certain fats tend to perpetuate the inflammatory response, keeping the body in a state of alarm. Conversely, diets rich in whole foods—colourful fruits and vegetables, healthy fats, lean proteins, whole grains—tend to calm it down. This big-picture understanding is the crux of what we call the 'diet-inflammation connection.'

Patterns Over Individual Foods

When trying to understand how diet influences inflammation, it helps to zoom out from just focusing on single foods or nutrients and focus on dietary patterns. Yes, certain foods such as leafy greens, oily fish, and berries are consistently heralded for their anti-inflammatory properties, and believe me we are going to be talking about these a lot. On the flip side processed meats, sugary drinks, and trans fats often appear on the pro inflammatory side of the spectrum. Yet, it is not always as simple as good food vs. bad food. Most people do not eat these items in isolation; they consume a combination of different foods every day, over many years. Just shovelling in a handful of blueberries is not going to negate a diet of kebabs and fizzy sweets. It is all about the whole picture.

That's why researchers frequently study 'dietary patterns'— general ways of eating that can be measured and analysed for broad effects on health. For instance, the Mediterranean diet, which emphasises whole grains, beans, vegetables, fruit, olive oil, fish, and moderate amounts of dairy, has been strongly correlated with lower levels of systemic inflammation. This style of eating provides an abundance of micronutrients, fibre, and beneficial fatty acids that, collectively, appear to soothe inflammatory processes. Many other traditional diets around the world (from East Asian diets built around vegetables, soy, and fish, to certain plant-forward African and South American cuisines) share similar features.

Compare this to the ultra-processed products and refined carbs typical of a modern Western pattern of eating. Such diets, often heavy in sugar-laden beverages, fried foods, and substantial amounts of red or processed meat, have been linked to higher levels of inflammatory markers. Often, these meals supply a surge of simple carbohydrates that spike blood sugar, as well as imbalanced ratios of certain fats that can promote inflammatory pathways. While a single indulgent meal here or there isn't going to ruin your health, a pattern of daily, long-term consumption is more likely to tilt your body towards chronic inflammation.

Linking Diet to Inflammatory Pathways

Although we are saving the nitty-gritty details of how various nutrients interact with inflammatory pathways for later chapters, it's useful to acknowledge the broad strokes here. One major factor is blood sugar control. There is a reason I talk about this so often, and even have a separate book on it. Spikes in blood glucose, often caused by consuming excessive refined sugars and processed carbs, can encourage the production of pro-inflammatory molecules within the body. Meanwhile, regularly consuming inadequate amounts of whole foods can deprive us of vitamins, minerals, antioxidants, and other beneficial compounds that help keep inflammation in check.

Beyond these micronutrients and the macronutrients like carbohydrates, protein, and fat, we also need to consider the importance of phytonutrients. These natural compounds, found predominantly in fruits, vegetables, herbs, and spices, often carry antioxidant properties that support a healthy inflammatory balance. Curcumin in turmeric, anthocyanins in berries, and polyphenols in olive oil are classic examples of compounds known to exhibit anti-inflammatory properties. When your plate is teeming with colourful, whole-food ingredients, it's easier to get a wide array of these protective substances.

However, it's not just about including the right foods; it's also about moderating or avoiding those with properties that may push the body towards unnecessary inflammation. An excess of refined seed oils, which are high in omega-6 fatty acids relative to omega-3s, can tip the balance. Overly salty, sweet, or artificial ingredients can also create metabolic stress. The resulting imbalance can be subtle at first, but cumulatively, over months and years, it encourages a low-level, chronic inflammatory state.

More Than Nutrients: The Role of Eating Behaviours

While the composition of your meals is crucial, how you eat and your relationship with food can also affect inflammation. Stress is a potent driver of inflammatory processes, and eating patterns often correlate closely with emotional states. Many people experience rushed meals, mindless snacking, or over-indulgences triggered by stress or fatigue. This can lead to a vicious cycle wherein poor food choices intensify stress on the body, which in turn can undermine self-control or mood, prompting further unwise dietary decisions.

Moreover, portion sizes have ballooned in many parts of the world, leading to overconsumption of energy-dense foods. Carrying excess weight, especially around the midsection, is itself associated with elevated levels of inflammation in the body. As weight increases beyond our healthiest range, fat cells (particularly visceral fat around the abdominal organs) produce signalling molecules that perpetuate inflammatory activity. This is part of why a balanced diet that supports a healthy body composition is so crucial for inflammatory health over the long term.

Timing also plays a role. Disrupted sleep patterns, for instance, can alter hormonal regulation of appetite, pushing you towards high-sugar or high-fat foods. A chaotic eating schedule—skipping meals, then bingeing later—can lead to large swings in blood sugar and stress hormones, again nudging the immune system towards imbalance. Although the key points about sleep, circadian rhythms, and other lifestyle factors will be explored later, it's important to see how these pieces fit together with your dietary choices to form a complete picture.

Large-scale population studies have given us a window into the diet-inflammation connection, often showing that people who consume diets rich in whole foods have lower levels of markers such as C-reactive protein (CRP), a common indicator of systemic inflammation. Conversely, high intakes of refined carbohydrates, sugary drinks, and processed meats have been associated with higher CRP levels.

Clinical trials have also helped demonstrate the effects of dietary changes. In some interventions, switching to a diet that emphasises fish, nuts, legumes, and vegetables—often in combination with moderate exercise and stress reduction—has yielded measurable reductions in inflammatory markers. Participants commonly report improvements in energy, mood, and even certain clinical symptoms. While not all trials agree on every nuance, the overall trend is that quality, minimally processed foods support a more balanced inflammatory response, and ultra-processed foods do the opposite.

Of course, correlation doesn't always imply causation, and humans are notoriously variable in their genetics, environments, and habits. One study might show remarkable results, while another detects only modest improvements. Yet, when researchers look at the totality of evidence, a consistent story emerges: the dietary pattern you adopt on a daily basis matters a great deal, and the changes you make don't have to be radical or painful to confer real benefits.

Though it's useful to understand the high-level science, day-to-day life is where the rubber meets the road. A truly anti-inflammatory approach involves taking stock of how your meals come together across the span of a week or month, rather than zeroing in on one 'perfect' day of eating or one occasional indulgence. It involves being mindful of ingredients when shopping, perhaps opting for fresh produce and whole grains over boxed or frozen meals with a long list of additives. It also involves reading labels more carefully—looking out for hidden sugars, refined oils, and artificial preservatives.

Importantly, it doesn't mean you can never enjoy a slice of cake or that you must banish favourite treats forever. Perfection is neither realistic nor required. Rather, the principle is about balance and consistency. If most of your meals feature wholesome, unprocessed foods that supply the nutrients your body needs, it becomes far less likely that the occasional indulgence will tip the scales towards chronic inflammation.

Once we have covered the science, I will take all of this information and actually translate it into something that you can use. A plan. With recipes and a practical framework you can use to build your anti-inflammatory diet in your day to day life.

PART 1:

UNDERSTANDING INFLAMMATION & IT'S IMPLICATIONS

I know you are here reading this book because you want to know how to change your diet to beat inflammation and start feeling better. But before we get into all of that, I need to set the stage. We need to have a bit of a science lesson so that you fully understand what is going on in your body. Not only does that keep you informed, it helps you to really know why I am making the recommendations that I am when it comes to the diet changes and enables you to make the right choices where ever you are. So lets start with looking at what inflammation is, how it works, and how it damages our health.

CHAPTER 1:
THE BIOLOGY OF INFLAMMATION

I hope you know me well enough by now to know that I want you to have the full picture. I am not about the superficial when it comes to my writing. Far too often in popular culture and media, the facts are diluted and glossed over. That does not serve you in any way shape or form does it? I believe that you need to be armed with as much information as possible in order to fully understand your health. This arms you perfectly to be able to do something about it. When you have all the facts and understand a subject fully, then you can get a better grasp on what you actually need to do.

So, its time to dive into some of the science. There may be parts that are a little complex, but I wanted to ensure that I have everything in here for you so that you can really get to grips with managing inflammation. Also, understanding all of these processes, enables you to really understand why I recommend that you make specific changes to your diet and build the dietary pattern that I recommend. You will be able to join the dots. This is the level of understanding I want to give you. So, lets dive in and take a look at how inflammation works and what physiological events take place when it happens. This will closely relate to the diet changes later on. All will become clear. I wont drag on forever as I know you are here for the diet plan, but stick with this section.

It's All About The Immune System

When we talk about inflammation, it is our immune system that really is the star of the show and the driving force behind everything. After all, the events we collectively label as 'inflammation' are mostly orchestrated by immune cells and the complex signalling networks they use. Yet, despite the enormous role the immune system plays in our daily health—whether defending against invaders or aiding in tissue repair—its everyday workings can sometimes be a mystery.

How Inflammation Begins

When a pathogen enters our body or breaches a barrier—say, bacteria entering a small cut on your skin—the local immune cells sense its presence via *pattern recognition receptors (PRRs)*. These are receptors that are capable of recognising certain chemical structures found on pathogens. When such things are detected, an alarm is raised and the troops are rallied.

In response, innate immune cells such as *macrophages* and *mast cells* release *inflammatory mediators* including histamine, prostaglandins, and cytokines. These mediators cause nearby blood vessels to dilate and become more permeable, allowing fluid, proteins, and additional white blood cells to flood the area—hence the classic signs of redness, heat, and swelling. This is *acute inflammation* in action. The reason these blood vessels expand and dilate is so that A) more blood and as such more white blood cells can be supplied to the area. And B) the dilation causes gaps to appear in the blood vessel walls. This allows white cells arriving in the area to squeeze through the gaps in the vessel walls and get to the area that needs assistance rapidly and effectively.

Innate responses then feed into adaptive immunity. If the threat persists, *antigen-presenting cells* (such as dendritic cells) process the offending material and travel to lymph nodes.

There, they display fragments of the pathogen on their surface. They put it on display, almost waving it around so it is noticed, effectively calling on T cells to initiate a more targeted assault. B cells, in turn, can produce specific antibodies that bind to the pathogen, marking it for destruction or neutralisation. This entire cascade of events shows how the immune system can rally an aggressive force quickly at first, then refine it for precision.

Tolerance and Regulation

A real key aspect of immune function is something known as *tolerance*. The immune system must distinguish between friend (self or beneficial external substance) and foe (non-self). If tolerance fails, we run the risk of autoimmune disorders, where the immune system begins attacking healthy tissues. Common autoimmune conditions would be rheumatoid arthritis and inflammatory bowel diseases. Specialised cells called *Regulatory T cells* (Tregs) play a significant role here, releasing cytokines (messenger proteins that carry messages between different cells and branches of the immune system) that restrict excessive immune activity and help to prevent pathological self-reactivity. IE autoimmunity.

The balance between effective defence and self-restraint from the immune system is delicate. Should the body overestimate threats or fail to dial down responses, inflammation can linger. This is where we start talking about 'chronic inflammation', a low-grade, ongoing process that can contribute to conditions such as arthritis, cardiovascular disease, and type 2 diabetes. Tolerance mechanisms and regulatory pathways are crucial for preventing such shifts into perpetual alarm mode.

Inflammation - a Symptom of Immune System Function

Although sometimes described as if it were something separate, inflammation is as we have seen really a by-product of immune activity. It represents both the body's attempt to eliminate harmful stimuli and the subsequent healing phase. In that sense, inflammation is like a red warning light on a car's dashboard. It signals that the immune system is switched on, doing its best to tackle a perceived problem. But if the immune system becomes confused or overstimulated—maybe the 'warning light' never switches off—it can start wearing down healthy tissue.

Acute inflammation is normally short-lived, often self-limiting as the immune system repairs the damaged area or clears the infection. Once the job is done, anti-inflammatory mediators and regulatory cells help restore the local environment. Chronic inflammation, however, lingers when the immune system either fails to eliminate the root cause or keeps misidentifying something harmless (like certain foods or even our own cells) as a threat. Or indeed lifestyle and environmental elements keep driving some of the key pathways involved. This can lead to the simultaneous presence of immune cells that both inflame and attempt to repair tissues, resulting in a destructive cycle that can last for months or even years.

One way chronic inflammation can take hold is through a communication breakdown in the immune system. If the balance of cytokines is disrupted—say, an overproduction of *TNF-alpha* and *IL-6* or an underproduction of *IL-10*—the body becomes stuck in an inflammatory state. Over time, this can generate a persistent 'background noise' of immune activation.

Autoimmune conditions often feature such breakdowns, where the immune system mistakes parts of the self for invaders. For example, in rheumatoid arthritis, immune cells attack the synovial lining of joints, causing swelling and pain. In type 1 diabetes, insulin-producing cells in the pancreas become the target. These misfires reflect a complex interplay between genetic susceptibility, environmental triggers (like infections or dietary factors), and immune regulation that has gone awry.

The Gut-Immune Axis

Though we will explore the gut's role in inflammation at length in a later chapter, it is important to note here that a large portion of the immune system is found in and around the gastrointestinal tract. This makes sense, as the gut is a major entry point for pathogens and foreign substances. Specialised tissues in the gut-associated lymphoid tissue (GALT) sample materials passing through the intestines, educating immune cells on what is harmful versus what is beneficial or neutral (like friendly bacteria or harmless food particles).

When the gut barrier is compromised—sometimes described as a 'leaky gut'—bacterial fragments or toxins can more easily pass into the bloodstream, triggering systemic immune responses. This often leads to low-grade, body-wide inflammation. Conversely, a healthy gut environment, supported by a balanced microbiome, can help maintain appropriate immune tolerance. This gut-immune interplay underpins why diet and inflammation are so tightly woven together and sets the stage for a wide range of interventions aimed at modulating immune responses through nutrition.

Understanding Inflammatory Mediators & Pathways

Another thing that you should understand are some of the molecules and pathways that drive inflammation. This doesn't need to get too complicated but this will really link directly to everything we discuss when it comes to diet, both in the positive and negative sense. Many nutritional components of the inflammatory picture link directly with these pathways and substances.

At the heart of the inflammatory processes are specific signalling pathways that coordinate how inflammation starts, what it does, and when it stops. These pathways are like carefully choreographed routines, designed to respond to threats and then return the body to balance. When these pathways function properly, they are our allies in healing and recovery. However, when they go haywire—becoming overactive or failing to resolve—they can lead to chronic inflammation and contribute to health problems.

The Role of Chemical Messengers

Inflammation relies heavily on chemical messengers that help immune cells communicate. We have seen that it is the immune system responding to stimuli that sets inflammation off, but it is the chemical messengers that direct the different cells and different branches of the immune system and tell them what to do when. These messengers tell the body when to start and stop an inflammatory response and coordinate which cells should respond. Among the most important of these are *cytokines, eicosanoids,* and other signalling molecules.

Cytokines: The Coordinators

Cytokines are small proteins that act like the body's internal communication system. They are produced by a wide variety of cells, including immune cells, and can have either *pro-inflammatory* or *anti-inflammatory* effects.

- **Pro-inflammatory cytokines**: These include molecules like *tumour necrosis factor-alpha (TNF-α), interleukin-1 beta (IL-1β),* and *interleukin-6 (IL-6)*. They are like alarms, calling immune cells to the site of injury or infection and ramping up the body's defences.

- **Anti-inflammatory cytokines**: These include *interleukin-10 (IL-10)* and *transforming growth factor-beta (TGF-β)*. They help resolve inflammation once the threat has been neutralised, ensuring the response doesn't go too far.

The balance between pro-inflammatory and anti-inflammatory cytokines is critical. Too much of the former can lead to chronic inflammation, while an overabundance of the latter may leave the body vulnerable to infections or slow healing. So many factors can affect this balance, especially lifestyle factors and even some infections themselves. Do you remember during COVID. many patients that had signs of metabolic illness - ie obesity, type 2 diabetes etc - were found to have far more serious effects from infection? Well, they already were in a state of chronic inflammation as that comes part and parcel with metabolic disease. When their bodies began fighting COVID, their pro-inflammatory cytokines ramped up even further and just kept going. This created what was referred to as a 'cytokine storm' which began causing untold damage to their body. These pathways need to work both ways effectively or it can really spell trouble.

The Eicosanoid Pathway

Eicosanoids are another group of key signalling molecules involved in inflammation. They are derived from fatty acids such as omega 3 and omega 6 (you will be hearing plenty more about these later) and include *prostaglandins, leukotrienes,* and *thromboxanes*. Eicosanoids play a central role in determining how intense and long-lasting an inflammatory response will be. These are going to be very familiar to you by the end of this book. Lets take a look at each:

Prostaglandins: The Amplifiers

Prostaglandins are produced at the site of injury or infection and are responsible for many of the classic symptoms of inflammation, including pain, swelling, and fever. They act on blood vessels to increase their permeability, allowing immune cells and other components to move into the affected area. They are also key players in reducing inflammation and reversing inflammation and resolving the situation. There has to be a balance between them or things can get out of control.

- Some prostaglandins promote inflammation, ensuring a robust response.

- Others help resolve inflammation by signalling when it's time to repair tissues and calm the immune system.

Leukotrienes: The Recruiters

Leukotrienes are another class of eicosanoids with a powerful role in inflammation. They are particularly active in conditions like asthma or allergies, where they help recruit immune cells to specific tissues. They beckon these key cells to the sites where they are needed and give them a nudge to deliver their unique specific benefits.

- They contribute to bronchoconstriction (narrowing of the airways), swelling, and increased mucus production in respiratory conditions.

- In other types of inflammation, leukotrienes help attract neutrophils and other immune cells to the site of damage.

Thromboxanes: The Clotters

Thromboxanes are involved in blood clotting and play a supporting role in inflammation. They help ensure that the site of injury is stabilised by promoting clot formation, which prevents further damage and seals the wound.

The above signalling molecules can be notably influenced by our diet, especially when it comes to fats and carbohydrates. All will become clear.

The NF-κB Pathway: The Master Switch

Ok, we do need to go a little bit deeper. One of the most important pathways in inflammation is the *NF-κB (nuclear factor kappa-light-chain-enhancer of activated B cells)* pathway. Bit of a mouthful I know. This pathway acts like a master switch, controlling the activation of many genes involved in the inflammatory response. Genes are the software that drives the hardware. The *NF-κB* pathway is the giant red switch that turns them on.

When the body detects an injury, infection, or other stress, NF-κB is activated in immune cells. Once switched on, it enters the cell's nucleus and activates relevant genes that trigger the production of cytokines, enzymes, and other inflammatory mediators. These molecules then set the inflammatory process in motion, recruiting immune cells and amplifying the response as needed.

The NF-κB pathway is essential for protecting the body, but its over activation has been linked to chronic inflammation. Conditions like rheumatoid arthritis, inflammatory bowel disease, and even some cancers have been associated with persistent NF-κB activity, which keeps the inflammatory response running long after it should have stopped.

The Inflammasome: A Critical Alarm System

The *inflammasome* is a multi-protein complex that serves as an alarm system within cells. It detects threats such as infections, toxins, or damaged cellular components and triggers the release of powerful inflammatory cytokines like IL-1β and IL-18.

The inflammasome's main job is to sense danger and initiate a rapid inflammatory response. For example, if a pathogen invades a cell or tissue damage releases debris, the inflammasome activates and helps recruit immune cells to the site. This process is crucial for clearing infections and repairing injuries.

Sometimes the inflammasome can be activated unnecessarily or remain active for too long. This inappropriate activation has been linked to chronic diseases such as type 2 diabetes, gout, and certain neurodegenerative disorders like Alzheimer's disease.

The Complement System

The *complement system* is another key player in inflammation. This group of proteins works in a cascade, like falling dominoes, to mark pathogens for destruction and assist immune cells in clearing infections. Complement proteins can:

- **Tag pathogens** for destruction by immune cells (a process called opsonisation).

- **Form membrane attack complexes**, which punch holes in cell walls of pathogens to kill them.

- **Recruit immune cells** to the site of infection or injury.

While the complement system is a critical defence mechanism, excessive or misdirected activation can cause tissue damage, contributing to autoimmune diseases and chronic inflammation.

Resolution: Turning Off Inflammation

Now this is a vital part of this whole picture. Active inflammation is one thing, but then what? Inflammation isn't meant to last forever. Once its job is done, the body has sophisticated mechanisms to resolve the response and promote healing. If inflammation were a fire, these mechanisms act as the firefighters, extinguishing the flames and ensuring no lasting damage. The resolution phase is as important as the initiation of inflammation. A well-functioning inflammatory response involves a swift and effective start, followed by an equally efficient resolution. Problems arise when this balance is disrupted—either because the initial response is too strong or because the resolution phase is delayed or incomplete. These factors again can be influenced by diet and lifestyle.

Specialised Pro-Resolving Mediators (SPMs)

SPMs are a group of molecules, including *resolvins, protec-tins,* and *maresins*, that actively turn off inflammation. These molecules signal immune cells to stop producing pro-inflammatory mediators and begin the process of tissue repair. Without SPMs, inflammation might persist unnecessarily, leading to chronic damage.

Biomarkers Of Inflammation

Before I jump to the next chapter where we will start to explore the impact that uncontrolled inflammation has on our health, you may well be interested in the types of tests that can be conducted to measure inflammation in your body and what each of these things actually are that could be measured on your doctors visit.

During an inflammatory episode, the body leaves behind measurable traces that help us understand what's happening under the surface. These traces, known as *biomarkers*, are substances produced or released in response to inflammation. They offer a glimpse into the immune system's activity, providing critical insights into both the intensity and type of inflammation present.

For someone experiencing chronic health issues or simply aiming to prevent them, understanding these biomarkers can be incredibly useful. They not only serve as diagnostic tools for clinicians but also act as indicators of how well inflammation is being managed.

What Are Biomarkers of Inflammation?

A biomarker is any measurable substance or parameter in the body that indicates a particular biological state. Biomarkers of inflammation specifically reflect the activity of the immune system and the processes driving inflammation. These markers can be proteins, molecules, or even specific cells found in blood, tissues, or other bodily fluids.

Inflammatory biomarkers are often divided into two broad categories:

1. **Acute-phase biomarkers**: Indicators of immediate, short-term inflammation, typically seen in response to infections or injuries.

2. **Chronic inflammation biomarkers**: Indicators of low-grade, persistent inflammation, often associated with long-term conditions like cardiovascular disease, diabetes, or autoimmune disorders.

By measuring these markers, clinicians can identify whether inflammation is present, determine its severity, and monitor the effectiveness of treatments or lifestyle changes.

The Key Biomarkers of Inflammation

1. C-Reactive Protein (CRP)

- **What it is**: CRP is a protein produced by the liver in response to inflammation. Its levels rise quickly during acute inflammation, making it a reliable marker for detecting sudden immune system activity.

- **Why it matters**: CRP is one of the most widely used inflammatory biomarkers because it's easy to measure through a blood test and provides a clear snapshot of systemic inflammation. Elevated CRP levels are commonly seen in infections, injuries, and chronic inflammatory conditions like rheumatoid arthritis or cardiovascular disease.

- **High-Sensitivity CRP (hs-CRP)**: A more refined version of the CRP test, hs-CRP is particularly useful for detecting low levels of chronic inflammation. It's often used to assess cardiovascular risk, as even mild increases in hs-CRP have been linked to heart disease and stroke.

2. Interleukin-6 (IL-6)

- **What it is**: IL-6 is a cytokine, or signalling protein, that plays a dual role in inflammation. It can both promote and regulate inflammatory responses depending on the context.

- **Why it matters**: IL-6 is often elevated in conditions involving chronic, systemic inflammation, such as type 2 diabetes, obesity, and autoimmune diseases. It also triggers the production of CRP in the liver, making it a key upstream player in the inflammatory cascade.

3. Tumour Necrosis Factor-Alpha (TNF-α)

- **What it is**: TNF-α is a powerful pro-inflammatory cytokine produced by immune cells like macrophages. It plays a central role in driving inflammation, particularly in autoimmune and inflammatory diseases.

- **Why it matters**: Elevated TNF-α levels are commonly found in rheumatoid arthritis, inflammatory bowel disease, and psoriasis. It is often a target for biologic therapies aimed at reducing excessive inflammation in these conditions.

4. Erythrocyte Sedimentation Rate (ESR)

- **What it is**: ESR is a measure of how quickly red blood cells settle at the bottom of a test tube. During inflammation, proteins like fibrinogen cause red blood cells to clump together, making them settle faster.

- **Why it matters**: ESR is a non-specific marker of inflammation that provides a general sense of whether inflammatory activity is present. While less precise than CRP, it is often used in conjunction with other tests to assess inflammatory conditions like lupus, arthritis, or infections.

5. Fibrinogen

- **What it is**: Fibrinogen is a blood-clotting protein that increases during inflammation. It plays a role in wound healing and tissue repair but can also contribute to excessive clot formation when levels are chronically elevated.

- **Why it matters**: High fibrinogen levels are associated with an increased risk of cardiovascular disease and other chronic conditions driven by inflammation.

6. Interleukin-1 Beta (IL-1β)

- **What it is**: IL-1β is another pro-inflammatory cytokine that acts as a key driver of inflammation, particularly in acute and autoimmune conditions. It is released in response to infections, injuries, and cellular stress.

- **Why it matters**: IL-1β plays a significant role in conditions like gout, where it contributes to joint inflammation, and in metabolic disorders like type 2 diabetes. It is also involved in the activation of the inflammasome, a key inflammatory complex.

7. Soluble Intercellular Adhesion Molecule-1 (sICAM-1)

- **What it is**: sICAM-1 is a molecule that helps immune cells adhere to the walls of blood vessels, allowing them to move into tissues where they're needed.

- **Why it matters**: Elevated levels of sICAM-1 are a marker of vascular inflammation and are associated with cardiovascular disease and metabolic syndrome.

8. Serum Amyloid A (SAA)

- **What it is**: SAA is another acute-phase protein produced by the liver during inflammation. It rises quickly in response to infection or injury, often alongside CRP.

- **Why it matters**: Persistently high levels of SAA are linked to chronic inflammatory conditions like arthritis, as well as increased cardiovascular risk.

What These Biomarkers Tell Us

Ok, so thats all well and good knowing what these things are, but what does that mean for you? Each of these biomarkers offers a different perspective on the inflammatory process. Some, like CRP and IL-6, provide a general overview of systemic inflammation, while others, like TNF-α or IL-1β, give more specific insights into the activity of certain pathways. By measuring these markers, doctors can:

1. **Identify Inflammation**: Determine whether inflammation is present, how severe it is, and whether it's acute or chronic.

2. **Pinpoint Underlying Causes**: Help narrow down potential causes, such as autoimmune disorders, infections, or metabolic imbalances.

3. **Monitor Progress**: Track changes over time to see if treatments or lifestyle changes are reducing inflammation.

Limitations of Biomarkers

While biomarkers provide valuable insights, they are not perfect. Many of them, like CRP and ESR, are **non-specific**, meaning they can indicate inflammation but don't necessarily reveal the exact cause. For example, elevated CRP might suggest an infection, an autoimmune flare, or even a transient response to exercise or stress.

Additionally, some biomarkers, such as cytokines, can fluctuate throughout the day or in response to factors like sleep, stress, or recent meals. This variability means that a single measurement is often less informative than trends observed over time.

Chronic vs. Acute Inflammation: What the Biomarkers Say

Acute inflammation is typically marked by sharp spikes in biomarkers like CRP, SAA, and IL-1β, reflecting the body's rapid response to a short-term threat. For example, after surgery or a bacterial infection, these markers might increase significantly but return to normal once healing is complete.

Chronic inflammation, on the other hand, often involves **low-grade, persistent elevations** in markers such as hs-CRP, IL-6, and TNF-α. This type of inflammation might not produce obvious symptoms at first, but over time, it can contribute to the development of diseases like type 2 diabetes, cardiovascular disease, or Alzheimer's.

Next time you have a blood test with your doctor or practitioner, you will have a clearer idea what some of this terminology actually means and it will help you gauge a true ides of where you are at personally.

CHAPTER 2:
THE IMPACT OF CHRONIC INFLAMMATION ON HEALTH

N ow we have an idea of what inflammation is and the key things that drive it, and we also know that chronic inflammation is the problematic variety, we need to explore how and why it damages our health and the links between chronic inflammation and common serious health complaints. Why is it even such a problem and why should we make any kind of effort at all to bring it under control?

As a persistent, low-grade state, chronic inflammation exerts systemic (whole body) effects, damaging tissues and disrupting normal physiological processes. This doesn't just affect the obvious things like our joints in arthritis. It is actually the driver for most of the degenerative diseases that fill our hospitals. The everyday conditions that we just accept as a 'thing' when we get older. The big killers and the conditions that drastically affect our quality of life. You may well be surprised when you see some of the conditions that it drives.

Metabolic Diseases

This is the big one. This is the one that cuts lives short. Metabolic diseases are the diseases that fill our wards and fill our doctors surgeries. When you take winter infections, accidents and acute emergencies out of the equation, what is it that fills our hospitals? Complications arising from type 2 diabetes, obesity, cardiovascular disease etc. These are all metabolic diseases and are a product of our lifestyle. This isn't to point the finger or to throw blame but these chronic conditions are becoming more and more common and are driven by the body's response to multiple negative environmental stimuli over time. It is pretty clear that our lifestyles, stress loads, diets, pollution exposure and more are a million miles away from what our bodies where designed to deal with. Even though the factors that trigger these conditions and cause them to develop in the first place, all of these metabolic issues share one common factor that drives their progression - chronic inflammation. It is inflammation that puts the foot on the gas and makes these conditions go from bad to worse.

Type 2 Diabetes

The prevalence of this is getting scary. There are over 3 and a half million people with type 2 diabetes in England alone. Way over 4 million for the entire UK. 2024 saw a 40% increase in young people too. I have seen children as young as FOUR in my clinic with the beginnings of type 2 diabetes. There is something very very wrong with how we are living here. In America it is even worse. 2024 data showed that there are over 38 million Americans with diabetes and 90-95% of these cases were type 2. This is unfathomable.

Type 2 diabetes (T2D) is a prime example of how chronic inflammation disrupts metabolic health. The condition is marked by *insulin resistance*, where cells fail to respond adequately to insulin, leading to elevated blood glucose levels. Chronic low-grade inflammation plays a direct role in the development of insulin resistance (Hotamisligil, 2006).

Insulin resistance often happens when there is prolonged elevated, unregulated blood sugar. But before that happens, other aspects of our metabolic health start to go South. We start to gain weight and our cardiovascular health takes a nose dive. This is because excess glucose will soon be sent to the liver where it is converted into triglycerides. These are fats that can be stored easily. They are created in the liver and then shipped off to our fat cells. Especially those around our middle. That causes abdominal weight gain. But, they are transported to the fat cells via our circulation, meaning that our blood fats go up and this damages cardiovascular health.

Adipose (fat) tissue, particularly visceral fat, is a significant source of inflammatory cytokines such as *tumour necrosis factor-alpha (TNF-a)* and *interleukin-6 (IL-6)*. These cytokines interfere with insulin signalling pathways by altering the function of insulin receptors, reducing the uptake of glucose into cells (Shoelson et al., 2006). This often also happens in individuals who are not obese too. A poor metabolic environment created by poor diet, lack of exercise and poor stress management can all have exactly the same impact so this is not unique to obese patients.

Elevated levels of *C-reactive protein (CRP)*, a marker of systemic inflammation, are consistently observed in individuals with insulin resistance or T2D (Pradhan et al., 2001). Chronic hyperglycaemia, in turn, creates a cycle of inflammation by generating *advanced glycation end-products (AGEs)* and oxidative stress, further exacerbating tissue damage. This cycle of events just keeps going on and on and on as the disease progresses. There is a key big change to make in this plan that will address these issues.

Obesity

Obesity is both a driver and consequence of chronic inflammation. Excessive adipose (fat) tissue, particularly visceral fat which is the type of fat that accumulates around our organs, acts as a hormonally active organ in its own right, releasing inflammatory mediators such as *TNF-a, IL-6*, and *monocyte chemoattractant protein-1 (MCP-1)* (Weisberg et al., 2003). These mediators attract immune cells like macrophages to adipose tissue, where they amplify the inflammatory response.

As fat cells expand (a condition known as hypertrophy), they can outgrow their blood supply, leading to cellular hypoxia (low oxygen levels). Hypoxia triggers the release of additional inflammatory signals and promotes the death of fat cells, further fuelling local and systemic inflammation (Ye, 2013). This chronic inflammatory state increases the risk of developing insulin resistance, T2D, cardiovascular disease, and non-alcoholic fatty liver disease (NAFLD). It becomes like a snowball.

Cardiovascular Disease

Cardiovascular disease (CVD) encompasses conditions like atherosclerosis, coronary artery disease, and stroke, all of which are strongly associated with chronic inflammation. Atherosclerosis, the build-up of plaques in arterial walls, is now understood as a chronic inflammatory disease rather than simply a lipid disorder (Libby, 2012).

Inflammation plays a central role at every stage of atherosclerosis. Low-density lipoprotein (LDL) cholesterol becomes oxidised within arterial walls, triggering an immune response. Macrophages engulf the oxidised LDL, forming foam cells that contribute to plaque formation. Cytokines and inflammatory enzymes released in the process promote further immune cell recruitment and destabilisation of plaques, increasing the risk of rupture and subsequent heart attack or stroke (Ridker et al., 2017). Elevated levels of CRP and IL-6 have been shown to predict cardiovascular events, emphasising the link between systemic inflammation and heart disease. Reduce the inflammation, reduce the risk.

Non-Alcoholic Fatty Liver Disease (NAFLD)

NAFLD, a condition characterised by the accumulation of fat in liver cells, has become a leading cause of liver-related deaths worldwide. Chronic inflammation is central to its progression, particularly in its more severe form, *non-alcoholic steatohep-*

atitis (NASH). Pro-inflammatory cytokines such as TNF-α and IL-6 contribute to liver cell injury, fibrosis, and eventual scarring (Tilg & Moschen, 2010). Over time this makes the liver less and less able to function and can lead to cirrhosis which is a life shortening condition.

Increased levels of inflammatory markers like CRP and adipokines (hormones released by fat tissue) are often observed in individuals with NAFLD, linking metabolic inflammation to liver dysfunction.

Well Known Chronic Inflammatory Diseases

Next we have the diseases that are more well known inflammatory conditions and that blight the lives of millions of people worldwide. The pain and discomfort that they cause is life altering and patients of these conditions are usually on multiple medications to deal with them. But what if we could change our diet in a way that enhances the activity of meciations and also leacs to prolonged relief and even dramatic improvement of the condition? Well, that is what this book is all about. So what diseases are we talking about here?

Rheumatoid Arthritis

Rheumatoid arthritis (RA) is a classic example of an autoimmune disorder driven by chronic inflammation. In RA, the immune system mistakenly attacks the synovial membranes of joints. This is like a soft tissue capsule that enshrouds the joint and holds everything in place. This targeting by the immune system leads to inflammation, swelling, and pain. Over time, this process damages cartilage and bone, causing joint deformity. Often we see what is called bilateral distribution, where both sides have the same type of distortion and deformity.

Key inflammatory mediators involved in RA include TNF-α, IL-1β, and IL-6, which drive the recruitment of immune cells and the destruction of joint tissues (Smolen et al., 2016). Treatments targeting these cytokines, such as TNF inhibitors, have revolutionised RA management, underscoring the importance of these pathways in disease progression. The beauty is, we can ramp this up even further with diet.

A note about osteoarthritis here. Whilst it has a different cause - ie it is wear and tear of the joints rather than the immune system destroying it, inflammation is still at its core in terms of the symptoms we feel. With that in mind all of the diet changes and principles that I will be outlining in this book will still be relevant if you suffer from OA.

Inflammatory Bowel Disease

Diseases in this spectrum are becoming more and more common. Alarming so in some populations. Inflammatory bowel disease (IBD), which includes *Crohn's disease* and *ulcerative colitis*, involves chronic inflammation of the gastrointestinal tract. While the exact causes remain unclear, an overactive immune response to gut microbes is thought to play a significant role. But what is it that influences the composition of our gut microbiome? It is of course our diet. Now, I am not saying that these issues are diet triggered, but by changing our diet and influencing the microbiome, plus adopting broad anti-inflammatory diet principles, we can change the picture.

In IBD, cytokines such as TNF-α and IL-17 drive inflammation, leading to symptoms like abdominal pain, diarrhoea, and weight loss. The chronic inflammation can also cause complications like erosion of the gut wall, fistulas, strictures, and a notable increased risk of colorectal cancer (Ungaro et al., 2017). Biomarkers like CRP and faecal calprotectin are often used to monitor disease activity.

Psoriasis

Most of the common skin complaints that plague us have an inflammatory component to them and following an anti-inflammatory diet will give notable improvement to any of them. The redness that comes with them and makes them look so obvious - that is inflammation. If we tackle that we can tackle the severity of the lesion.

Psoriasis is one of the most aggressive and is a chronic inflammatory condition marked by the rapid turnover of skin cells and the formation of red, scaly patches. The immune system plays a central role, with overactive T cells releasing cytokines like *IL-17, IL-23*, and *TNF-α*, which drive inflammation and abnormal skin cell growth (Lowes et al., 2014).

Psoriasis is also linked to systemic inflammation, increasing the risk of comorbidities such as cardiovascular disease and metabolic syndrome.

In skin issues such as acne and eczema, that redness that comes at the beginning of a flare up or outbreak. The red patches that start an eczema flare up or the raised red bump in an acne breakout. That is inflammation. If we target inflammation then we can make those types of skin lesions look less severe. The redness and irritation and pain is less severe. Regulating inflammation is a key part of managing these skin conditions too.

Asthma

Asthma is a chronic respiratory condition characterised by inflammation of the airways, leading to symptoms like wheezing, coughing, and shortness of breath. Inflammatory mediators such as leukotrienes, IL-4, and IL-13 are key drivers of airway inflammation, hyper responsiveness, and mucus production (Barnes, 2008). This is a condition that features flare ups and 'attacks' when the immune system becomes over responsive to a specific stimuli. Asthma, eczema and hay fever are actually all the same condition, they just manifest in different tissues. They are type 2 hypersensitivity reactions where the immune system responds to a specific stimuli - dust mites, pollen etc, but the response is completely over the top and beyond what is necessary, and causes inflammation to go out of control.

Chronic inflammation in asthma can result in airway remodelling, causing long-term damage and reduced lung function. Effective treatments, including corticosteroids and leukotriene receptor antagonists, aim to reduce inflammation and prevent exacerbations.

Neurodegenerative Diseases & Depression

The next group of diseases I want to talk about are a group that normally we would never associate with inflammation, but new research is showing have a strong and consistent inflammatory component. That is neurodegenerative diseases and depression. The inflammatory link here may surprise you. However, when we think about the rising prevalence of such conditions, and the lifestyle factors that drive inflammation, it really is not that surprising.

Alzheimer's Disease

Emerging evidence suggests that chronic inflammation contributes significantly to the development of Alzheimer's disease (AD). The accumulation of amyloid-beta plaques and tau tangles in the brain triggers activation of the microglia (resident immune cells of our brain), leading to the release of pro-inflammatory cytokines such as IL-1β and TNF-α. This neuroinflammatory response exacerbates neuronal damage and accelerates cognitive decline (Heneka et al., 2015). When you think about it, many of the alzheimers risk factors - alcohol consumption, poor diet, prolonged stress etc are all things that trigger and exacerbate inflammation. Could this be why they are risk factors in the first place?

Parkinson's Disease

In Parkinson's disease (PD), chronic inflammation in the brain is thought to contribute to the loss of dopaminergic neurons. Elevated levels of inflammatory cytokines, as well as increased activation of microglia, have been observed in affected individuals (Hirsch & Hunot, 2009). Chronic systemic inflammation may also play a role, with studies linking elevated CRP levels to an increased risk of PD.

Depression

This is one that may surprise you. There are now links between depression and neuroinflammation. Chronic, low-grade inflammation can alter brain function in ways that promote depressive symptoms. Elevated levels of inflammatory markers, including *C-reactive protein (CRP)*, *interleukin-6 (IL-6)*, and *tumour necrosis factor-alpha (TNF-α)*, have been consistently observed in individuals with depression (Miller & Raison, 2016). Moreover, treatments that reduce inflammation, such as anti-inflammatory medications, have shown promise in alleviating depressive symptoms in some cases (Köhler et al., 2014).

Key mechanisms linking neuroinflammation to depression include:

1. **Cytokine Signalling**: Pro-inflammatory cytokines can cross the blood-brain barrier or signal the brain indirectly, activating microglia and astrocytes (specialised immune cells in the brain). This activation leads to further release of inflammatory molecules, creating a feedback loop that sustains neuroinflammation.

2. **Altered Neurotransmission**: Neurotransmitters are chemical messengers in the brain that regulate everything from moving our limbs, to sleep patterns and even our mood. Inflammation affects the synthesis, release, and reuptake of key neurotransmitters such as serotonin, dopamine, and glutamate. Pro-inflammatory cytokines like IL-6 and TNF-α

can disrupt serotonin production by increasing the activity of the enzyme *indoleamine 2,3-dioxygenase (IDO)*, which diverts tryptophan (a precursor to serotonin) into the kynurenine pathway, reducing serotonin availability (Capuron & Miller, 2011).

3. **Neuroplasticity Impairment**: Chronic inflammation can inhibit the production of *brain-derived neurotrophic factor (BDNF)*, a protein essential for neurogenesis and synaptic plasticity. Reduced BDNF levels are strongly associated with depression and impaired cognitive function (Dowlati et al., 2010).

4. **HPA Axis Dysregulation**: Inflammatory signals can dysregulate the *hypothalamic-pituitary-adrenal (HPA) axis*, leading to elevated cortisol levels. Chronic cortisol release further promotes inflammation, creating a vicious cycle that exacerbates depressive symptoms.

Cancer

Then finally we have the big elephant in the room. This is not hyperbole or an outlandish claim. Look in any A level or high school pathology text book and you will see that it is a well established fact that prolonged inflammation can lead to cellular changes that trigger cancer. Firstly, the inflammation can affect genes within the cells. Specifically genes that regulate the rate and extent to which cells divide. If this changes then cellular division can get out of control and tumour formation can begin.

Chronic inflammation is now recognised as a key factor in cancer development. Inflammatory cytokines such as IL-6, TNF-α, and IL-1β promote tumour growth by increasing cell proliferation, suppressing apoptosis (programmed cell death), and stimulating the formation of new blood vessels (angiogenesis) (Colotta et al., 2009). Once angiogenesis occurs, tumours can begin to flourish rapidly.

Certain inflammatory conditions, such as chronic hepatitis (linked to liver cancer) or ulcerative colitis (linked to colorectal cancer), demonstrate how persistent inflammation can create an environment conducive to cancer development.

CHAPTER 3:

THE NON DIETARY LIFESTYLE DRIVERS OF CHRONIC INFLAMMATION

The bulk of this book is, of course, dedicated to the role of diet in inflammation and how we can adapt our diets to be an anti-inflammatory powerhouse. That is coming. But before we dive into the food, we need to take a long, hard look at the other lifestyle factors that are driving chronic inflammation. These are the things that have become so normal in our daily lives that we barely even notice them anymore. They are the silent instigators, constantly fanning the flames of inflammation. If we ignore them, we are missing half the picture. Covering this now allows us to make conscious decisions to improve behaviours, take control, and set ourselves up for success before we even get to the food. And there's an added bonus. Many of these lifestyle factors overlap with diet. The two are intertwined in ways that might not be immediately obvious, and by understanding them, we can use food strategically to influence them. This is about layering multiple defences, stacking the odds in our favour, and creating an environment where inflammation is not just reduced—it's crushed.

Let's start with stress. There is no getting away from it. Modern life is relentless. We are living so far removed from the environment our bodies evolved for that we are in a constant battle with our own physiology. Our still-primitive survival mechanisms, designed to keep us out of danger, are being activated dozens of times a day. Family pressures, financial worries, work stress, the chaos of the daily commute, social media anxiety, and the ever-present stream of negative news. It's an all-out assault on our nervous system. And the result? Chronic, low-grade stress that never really switches off.

Now, stress in itself isn't inherently bad. It's a survival mechanism. When we perceive a threat, our body releases cortisol, a stress hormone that increases glucose availability and raises blood pressure—preparing us to fight or flee. That's fine if we're running from a sabre-toothed tiger. But when the "threat" is an overflowing inbox or a passive-aggressive email, the stress response is doing us far more harm than good. The real issue comes when this stress is prolonged or repeated, causing the body's stress response system, the hypothalamic-pituitary-adrenal (HPA) axis, to become dysregulated. When this happens, cortisol loses its ability to regulate inflammation properly. Instead of dampening down inflammatory responses, it begins to malfunction, leading to a rise in pro-inflammatory cytokines—molecules that drive inflammation (Furman et al., 2019). Research has consistently linked chronic stress to elevated levels of inflammatory markers such as interleukin-6 (IL-6) and tumour necrosis factor-alpha (TNF-α), both of which are associated with conditions ranging from cardiovascular disease to depression and autoimmune disorders (Slavich & Irwin, 2014). The science is clear: stress is not just an emotional state. It's a biochemical event with real, measurable physiological consequences.

And then there's sleep. Sleep is something we all know we need more of, but modern life makes it increasingly difficult to prioritise. The problem is that sleep is not just about feeling rested. It is one of the most critical regulators of our immune system and inflammatory control. While we sleep, the body releases anti-inflammatory compounds, repairs tissues, and carries out essential immune functions. When we skimp on sleep, we disrupt these processes, leading to higher levels of inflammatory markers. Poor sleep is directly associated with increased C-reactive protein (CRP), a key indicator of systemic inflammation (Irwin, 2015).

But it gets worse. Our immune system follows a circadian rhythm, meaning it operates on a 24-hour cycle, responding to different triggers at different times of the day. When our sleep patterns are erratic—due to shift work, late-night screen use, or stress—our immune function gets thrown off balance. This is why shift workers, whose sleep cycles are chronically disrupted, have a much higher risk of inflammatory diseases, including type 2 diabetes, heart disease, and even certain cancers (Cedernaes et al., 2019). Sleep deprivation doesn't just leave us feeling groggy. It actively fuels the inflammatory fire.

And what about movement? Humans are built to move. For most of our evolution, we spent our days in constant motion—hunting, gathering, building, and travelling on foot. Our bodies adapted to this high level of activity. But modern life has made us sedentary. Many of us spend hours sitting at a desk, commuting in cars, and then collapsing onto the sofa at the end of the day. It's a recipe for disaster.

Physical inactivity is one of the most potent yet overlooked drivers of inflammation. When we don't move enough, visceral fat accumulates—the kind of fat that wraps around our organs and secretes inflammatory molecules like TNF-α and IL-6. At the same time, our production of anti-inflammatory molecules, such as interleukin-10 (IL-10), plummets. This imbalance puts us at greater risk of everything from metabolic syndrome to neurodegenerative disease (Beavers et al., 2010).

The good news? Exercise is one of the most powerful anti-inflammatory tools we have. Even a single bout of moderate-intensity exercise has been shown to reduce inflammation, triggering a cascade of beneficial effects that lower pro-inflammatory cytokines and boost anti-inflammatory defences (Gleeson et al., 2011). Regular physical activity doesn't just help maintain a healthy weight. It actively alters our immune system, reducing systemic inflammation and enhancing metabolic health.

But let's take it a step further. Beyond stress, sleep, and movement, we also have to acknowledge the role of environmental toxins. This is an area that is both controversial and, frankly, under-discussed. Our modern environment is packed with chemicals that were never part of human evolution, and many of them have direct inflammatory effects.

Air pollution is one of the biggest culprits. We breathe in tiny particulate matter that penetrates deep into our lungs, enters the bloodstream, and sparks systemic inflammation. Research has linked air pollution exposure to increased inflammatory markers, cardiovascular disease, and even neurodegenerative conditions like Alzheimer's (Brook et al., 2010). Then we have endocrine-disrupting chemicals (EDCs)—synthetic compounds found in plastics, pesticides, and industrial products. These chemicals interfere with hormonal regulation, increasing inflammation and altering immune function (Patisaul & Adewale, 2009).

And then there's the issue of heavy metals. Lead, mercury, and cadmium accumulate in the body over time, activating inflammatory pathways and causing damage at a cellular level. Chronic exposure to these toxins has been associated with autoimmune disorders, cardiovascular disease, and cognitive decline (Tchounwou et al., 2012).

The takeaway from all of this? Inflammation is not just about food. It is influenced by every aspect of our modern lives. Stress, sleep, movement, and environmental exposure all play a role in driving or reducing inflammation. The good news is that we can take control. By managing stress, prioritising sleep, staying active, and minimising exposure to environmental toxins, we can create a foundation that supports our body's ability to regulate inflammation. And when we combine these lifestyle changes with the right diet? That's when we unlock the full potential of an anti-inflammatory lifestyle.

CHAPTER 4:
THE GUT INFLAMMATION CONNECTION

The gut is not just a digestive organ. Far from it. It is an active, dynamic, and highly complex interface between the external environment and the body's internal systems. It is at the very heart of immune function and inflammatory regulation. It stands as the body's first line of defence, constantly interacting with food, microbes, and environmental compounds, deciding what is safe and what must be attacked. And when this system goes wrong? Well, that's when things can spiral out of control, leading to systemic inflammation, metabolic disorders, autoimmune diseases, and a cascade of health issues that seem to come out of nowhere (Cani et al., 2007).

Two major aspects of gut health play a pivotal role in inflammation: the microbiome and the integrity of the gut barrier. When these two systems are in harmony, inflammation is well-regulated, and the body maintains balance, or what we call homeostasis. But when they are disturbed—when the microbiome is thrown into chaos or the gut barrier becomes leaky—the consequences can be catastrophic (Fasano, 2012).

Now, let's talk about the microbiome. This is not some minor feature of human biology; it is a vast and intricate ecosystem teeming with trillions of bacteria, fungi, viruses, and other microscopic life forms, all living in the gastrointestinal tract. These microbes are not just passive hitchhikers, floating around in the gut doing nothing. They are active participants in digestion, metabolism, immunity, and, critically, the regulation of inflammation. They produce compounds that can either calm inflammation down or send it into overdrive. The problem? Modern life is doing its absolute best to wreck this delicate balance (Turnbaugh et al., 2006).

A healthy microbiome is diverse. It has an array of beneficial bacteria that keep potential troublemakers in check. But when this balance is lost—a state called dysbiosis—harmful microbes can take over, triggering immune activation and setting off chronic inflammation that doesn't just stay in the gut. It spreads. It affects the skin, the joints, the brain—no system is immune (Kostic et al., 2014).

One of the most important ways gut bacteria influence inflammation is through the production of short-chain fatty acids, or SCFAs. You've probably heard of these. They include butyrate, acetate, and propionate, and they are produced when gut bacteria ferment dietary fibre. Now, butyrate is a bit of a superstar. It directly supports the gut lining, keeping it strong and intact. It also dials down pro-inflammatory cytokine production, keeping the immune system from going into overdrive. And if that wasn't enough, it promotes the production of regulatory T cells—cells that tell the immune system to calm the hell down when it's getting too aggressive. Without enough SCFAs, inflammation starts creeping up, slowly but surely (Furusawa et al., 2013).

But that's not all. The gut microbiota also metabolises tryptophan, an amino acid, into molecules that interact with immune cells in ways that further modulate inflammation. There are also bile acids, which the gut bacteria modify to regulate cytokine production and immune responses. So, the microbiome is constantly fine-tuning the immune system, keeping it responsive but not reckless (Agus et al., 2018).

But what happens when dysbiosis takes hold? The answer is simple: chronic inflammation. The balance shifts. Harmful bacteria start to produce pro-inflammatory compounds, immune cells get overstimulated, and the body enters a state of persistent immune activation. This isn't just a minor issue; it's a fundamental shift in health, linked to inflammatory bowel disease, metabolic disorders, and autoimmune conditions like rheumatoid arthritis and multiple sclerosis (López et al., 2021).

And then, of course, there's the issue of the gut barrier, the physical and biochemical boundary that separates the gut contents from the bloodstream. The intestinal lining is just a single cell layer thick. That's it. One layer of cells, held together by tight junctions, preventing unwanted substances from leaking into circulation. It is incredibly effective—when it works properly. But when this barrier becomes compromised, we have a problem. A big problem (Fasano, 2011).

This is what people refer to as 'leaky gut.' It means that the tight junctions between gut cells have weakened, allowing large molecules, bacterial fragments, and toxins to pass through into the bloodstream. The result? The immune system goes into a frenzy. It sees these foreign invaders where they shouldn't be and mounts an inflammatory response. Not just a mild, temporary response—this is chronic, systemic inflammation that never really shuts off. The more this happens, the worse things get (Cani et al., 2007).

One of the most notorious culprits in this process is lipopolysaccharide, or LPS. This is a molecule found on the outer membrane of certain bacteria, and when it gets into the bloodstream, it sends an alarm signal to the immune system that screams, 'Attack!' The problem? This attack doesn't just happen once. If the gut barrier is leaky, LPS continuously seeps into circulation, bombarding immune cells, triggering inflammatory cytokine production, and creating a state of chronic, low-grade inflammation. This is not just a theoretical concept—it is a measurable, well-documented phenomenon known as metabolic endotoxemia, and it is a major driver of type 2 diabetes, cardiovascular disease, and non-alcoholic fatty liver disease (Cani et al., 2007).

Leaky gut doesn't just impact metabolic health. It has also been linked to autoimmune diseases, where the immune system mistakenly attacks the body's own tissues. When the gut barrier weakens, bacterial antigens slip through into circulation, triggering an immune response that can lead to conditions like rheumatoid arthritis, lupus, and Hashimoto's thyroiditis (Fasano, 2012). And the effects don't stop there. Chronic gut-derived inflammation has been implicated in neurological disorders, including depression, anxiety, and even Alzheimer's disease. The gut and brain are in constant communication, and when inflammation starts in the gut, the brain feels the impact (Cryan & Dinan, 2012).

So, how do we fix this? How do we restore balance to the gut and reduce this chronic inflammation? The good news is that it is possible. The first step is to repair the gut barrier. This requires key nutrients like zinc, glutamine, and vitamins A and D, all of which support the integrity of the gut lining. But reducing stress is just as important. Chronic stress and high cortisol levels wreak havoc on the gut barrier, making everything worse. Mindfulness practices, breathwork, and stress management techniques can go a long way in calming the gut and reducing inflammation (Fasano, 2011).

And then there's the microbiome. This needs to be restored, rebalanced, and supported. Eating a diverse, fibre-rich diet is the best way to encourage the growth of beneficial microbes. Prebiotics—fibres that feed good bacteria—are essential, as are probiotics, which introduce beneficial bacteria directly into the gut. Antibiotic overuse needs to be minimised. While they are sometimes necessary, antibiotics wipe out entire bacterial populations, leaving the microbiome vulnerable to dysbiosis and inflammation (Turnbaugh et al., 2006).

The gut's role in inflammation is profound. It is not just about digestion. It is a highly intelligent system, deeply connected to immune function, metabolic regulation, and overall health. When the microbiome is thriving, and the gut barrier is strong, inflammation is controlled, and the body maintains balance. But when these systems are disrupted, inflammation becomes chronic, and disease follows. Understanding this is the key to not just reducing inflammation but preventing a whole host of chronic diseases that seem to plague modern society.

PART 2:

HOW OUR DIET INFLUENCES INFLAMMATION

Now it is time for the bit you have been waiting for. How our food influences this whole picture and what you can actually do about it. There is a lot that we are going to go through here as I am all bout you having a broad understanding of everything so that you actually know why you are doing what I recommend that you do. The good news is though, the actual day to day 'plan' ie the changes to your diet that you will make are actually very simple. Not to mention delicious.

CHAPTER 5:
THE FOODS THAT FUEL THE FIRE

There are some foods that we consume far to regularly that are to inflammation what petrol is to a bonfire. Foods that drive inflammation and affect how aggressively it develops. Unfortunately, these are the foods that have dominated our diet for several decades since we became more and more reliant upon processed foods and convenience. The further we move from the food we are designed to eat, the worse this pattern gets. So before we look at the food that can actually turn this picture around, I want to explain why many of the foods that have become commonplace in our modern diets are actually making things worse. Which will be exactly why I recommend you avoid them.

Refined Carbohydrates & Simple Sugars

Probably not a huge shock here, but this is a vital place to start. Most of us are aware that too much sugar and processed carbohydrate isn't good for us, but fewer people realise just how deeply refined carbohydrates and sugars impact inflammation. These foods have become ever more prevalent in our modern diets. Years ago we would only eat brown bread. In most parts of Asia, brown rice was the norm until someone convinced people that the 'polished' white version (the same grain with the outer husk removed) was a better option. We have abandoned beautiful health giving foods to allow for their highly refined and dangerous versions.

The good news? Once we understand how refined carbs and sugars trigger inflammation, we can make simple but powerful changes that significantly reduce our risk of long-term health problems.

Carbohydrates come in many different forms, some of which are beneficial, and others that can be harmful when eaten in excess.

Refined carbohydrates are processed foods that have been stripped of their fibre, vitamins, and minerals, leaving behind only fast-digesting starches and sugars. These foods flood your bloodstream with sugar quickly, causing spikes in blood glucose that set off a chain reaction of inflammatory processes.

The Worst Offenders: Inflammatory Carbohydrates

These are the foods that rapidly break down into sugar in the body, driving inflammation:

- **White bread, white rice, and white pasta** (refined grains)

- **Pastries, cakes, and biscuits etc** (high in both sugar and refined flour)

- **Sugary cereals** (often marketed as 'healthy' but packed with sugar)

- **Soft drinks and fruit juices** (liquid sugar that hits the bloodstream fast)

- **Processed snacks like crackers and granola bars**

- **Flavoured yoghurts** (even low-fat versions are loaded with sugar)

- **Sauces, dressings, and condiments** (many contain hidden sugars)

These foods provide quick energy but little nutrition, and over time, they disrupt blood sugar levels, trigger weight gain, and keep the body in a constant state of inflammation. They fan the flame.

When you eat refined carbohydrates such as the ones listed above, your blood sugar levels shoot up quickly because there is no fibre to slow digestion. Foods like white rice and white bread do not contain any more glucose than their whole grain versions. The issue is the lack of fibre. This means that the glucose content is liberated rapidly. Instead of a gentle trickle, blood sugar is carpet bombed and that is the issue. The speed and extent to which blood sugar rises within a short window and the hormonal and physical response that takes place when this happens. In response to the sugar spike, your body releases a surge of insulin, a hormone that helps move sugar out of the bloodstream and into cells.

This might not seem like a big deal, and now and again it isn't but over time, constant blood sugar spikes can start to activate some key inflammatory events. Firstly dysregulated blood glucose can trigger pro-inflammatory pathways that release inflammatory chemicals like TNF-α, IL-6, and CRP (Esposito et al., 2002). If other events have already activated these pathways, this additional onslaught will make matters far worse and start that inflammatory snowball rolling.

Now and again this kind of blood sugar roller coaster is no big deal. However, if it goes on for a long time, then things can start to go wrong and the damage sets in. Firstly, the body stores more fat, particularly around the belly, where it releases inflammatory chemicals. This is because the excess sugar is turned into fat to make it easier to get out of the way and be stored where it is less harmful in the immediate sense. Blood sugar cannot get too high or too low. Either state is potentially life threatening, so the body has very effective ways of responding to each situation. When blood sugar rises, the body responds by releasing the hormone insulin. This tells our cells that blood sugar has risen above the set limit and there is some available for them to use as energy, so they need to open the doors and let some glucose in. All well and good. The thing is, our cells can only take in so much glucose in one single sitting. Too much can cause them damage so once they are full they close the doors and do not let any more glucose in. When this happens, if blood glucose is still above the threshold, it still has to be dealt with. The body's next trick is to convert some of that glucose into something called glycogen. This is a storage form of glucose that is stored in the liver and in our muscles. The problem is, there is only so much glycogen our body can store. Now, in most situations, these two responses would be enough. If however we are following the typical Western diet of highly refined carbohydrates and processed sugary foods, then we are easily able to raise our blood glucose to a stage where it goes beyond the point that our cells and glycogen can deal with it. If our cells are full and glycogen stores are at capacity, then any excess glucose still has to be dealt with. It has to go somewhere as that excess circulating glucose can cause a great deal of damage to tissues by means of glucotoxicity. At this stage, the excess glucose will be sent to the liver and in a chemical process called de novo lipogenesis, it will be converted into triglycerides, A form of storable fat which will then get sent to our adipose (fat) tissue. This gets it in storage out of the way so that it can no longer cause any damage and also can be used as a convenient energy source on a day when food is scarce. this is how we were designed to work during our evolution. How often do we experience that level of food scarcity today? Most people never get the chance to liberate any of that stored fat. This accumulation of fat during this process also tends to be visceral fat rather than subcutaneous. This visceral fat is the type that clings to your organs and that pumps out huge amounts of inflammatory chemicals. We need to avoid this pattern.

The good news does not stop there! If this pattern of excessive blood glucose continues over long periods, things take a far worse turn. When blood sugar is constantly high, the body produces more and more insulin. Eventually, the cells stop responding properly to the signals that insulin is sending, leading to insulin resistance—the first step towards type 2 diabetes, weight gain, and chronic inflammation (Shoelson et al., 2006).

As insulin resistance develops, many aspects of our physiology and metabolic health begin to get negatively affected.Inflammation worsens, making it even harder for insulin to work properly. This makes the whole process accelerate. The pancreas overworks itself, trying to keep up, leading to metabolic dysfunction.

Gut Damage: How Sugar Feeds Inflammation

As we saw in the last chapter, your gut is absolutely central to inflammation—it's where much of your immune system lives. The bacteria in your gut (your microbiome) control how much inflammation is happening inside your body. We covered that so I wont go over old ground, but what we need to realise is that to avoid the events covered in the last part of the book, we need to create an environment that supports a healthy microbiome and gut tissue. Most of that will come from the food that we eat. One of the worst contenders for damaging gut health - you guessed it. refined carbohydrates.

Refined carbs and sugars feed harmful bacteria, causing an imbalance (dysbiosis). If problematic bacteria get the upper hand - further inflammation and gut damage occur. Simple sugars are a convenient food source for these potentially dysbiotic organisms. Simple and refined carbohydrates also have the capacity to reduce beneficial bacteria that produce anti-inflammatory compounds like short-chain fatty acids (SCFAs). These substances maintain the health of the gut lining and barrier function and create a favourable environment for the flourishing of beneficial bacteria. Finally refined carbohydrates can in and of themselves damage the gut lining, allowing toxins and bacteria to enter the bloodstream (leaky gut), triggering widespread inflammation (Cani et al., 2007).

Advanced Glycation End Products (AGEs)

Now this is an interesting one and something seldom talked about in the mainstream. Excess sugar in the bloodstream binds to proteins, forming harmful molecules called *Advanced Glycation End Products (AGEs)*. AGEs are harmful compounds formed when refined carbohydrates rapidly raise blood sugar levels, leading to excessive glycation—where sugars bind to proteins and fats in the body. AGEs trigger oxidative stress, damaging cells and tissues and causing an inflammatory tidal wave. They also promote stiffening of blood vessels, increasing heart disease risk. The stiffer the vessels, the less resilient they are to fluctuations in blood pressure which can eventually increase the risk of vessel damage - setting the scene for heart disease and cardiovascular events. AGE's also Activate inflammation through the RAGE receptor. The Receptor for Advanced Glycation End Products (RAGE) is a cell surface receptor that binds to AGEs, triggering inflammatory and oxidative stress responses worsening conditions like arthritis and Alzheimer's disease (Vlassara & Striker, 2011).

Trans Fats and Omega-6-Rich Oils

Ok, if you know my work you are familiar with this soap box. The influence that the fats we consume has upon inflammation. Fats are a crucial part of our diet, but not all fats are created equal. There are some that offer huge benefit and there are some that are incredibly damaging. While some fats are anti-inflammatory and essential for health, others fuel chronic inflammation, increasing the risk of heart disease, obesity, autoimmune conditions, and even brain disorders.

Two of the biggest offenders? Trans fats and excess omega-6 fats from processed vegetable oils. These fats disrupt the body's balance, triggering inflammatory pathways, damaging cells, and contributing to chronic disease.

Trans fats have their own unique issues which I will discuss in a moment, but there is a bigger issue in the room. Our intake of omega 6 rich fats. These include things like vegetable oil, sunflower oil, soy bean oil etc. We are consuming vast amounts of these. But why? Why are there so many of them in our diet? Well, this is due to a series of events that took place about 50 years ago, in the form of a very ill informed public health campaign, sparked by the work of one man, named Ansel Keys. Keys was an American physiologist with a strong interest in nutrition. He had been part of many dietary projects with the US government, including the development of the K ration - a nutrient dense bar that was given to American troops in the field to give them daily sustenance, and full daily nutritional needs in a small portable unit. During his career, Keys had developed a theory that cardiovascular disease was caused by saturated fat and a nations heart disease statistics would be a direct reflection of the amount of saturated fat that the population ate. So, he set about to prove this. To do this he devised what was initially called 'The 22 Countries Study. The study literally was as it sounds - a study into the dietary habits of 22 countries. The intakes of saturated fat was compared against cardiovascular disease rates to search for the connection. Once the study was finished, the findings were published, and boy did they prove the saturated fat and heart disease hypothesis perfectly. case dismissed....or was it? The only problem was that the data published was from only 6 of the 22 countries. Hang on a second!!! 6? What happened to the rest? Well, if the data from all 22 countries were published, Keys' theory would have completely fallen apart. The full data set showed ABSOLUTELY NO CONNECTION at all between saturated fat intake and heart disease. But, Keys was an ambitious chap, and also had a lot of investment and backing that were certainly...keen...to see a specific result. So, the data was selected that showed what Keys wanted to show. He used the data from countries where a connection could be found, and that would support his ideas, and completely threw out the rest! This outright fraud should have been a massive news and scandal, but no. Keys became a national Hero, and in no time at all was on the front cover of Time magazine, and was beginning to advise on government public health policy. When this happened the US government soon developed a public health campaign that warned the American public to drastically reduce their intake of saturated fats. The same messaging came over to the UK within weeks too and a whole new view of diet and health was born. This farce caused an international public health campaign that drummed it into us that we need to avoid saturated fat like the plague, and instead opt of more 'heart healthy' options such as sunflower oil, vegetable oil, corn oil, soy oil - and the most hideous creations of all, margarine's etc. We were told to consume those because, you know, they were not saturated fats so they must be 'heart healthy'. That my friends is where things went very wrong indeed.

But, why would this actually be a problem? Well, these types of oils are made up almost completely of something called omega 6 fatty acids. Let's back track a moment. Fatty acids are fat derived, almost vitamin like substances that play a wide range of roles in the body from structural roles, such as building cell membranes, through to communication roles. It is the latter that is the issue. There are two essential fatty acids that our body needs to get from the diet, and are vital to health. Essential means that we cannot manufacture them from something else. We need to get them from dietary sources. These are omega 3 and omega 6 fatty acids. Both vital for health. If they are so important for health, whats the problem with those oils mentioned above? Well, omega 6 is only needed in very small amounts. When consumed in these small amounts it plays some very important roles in our body. But, once we get past this amount in a day, this once beneficial compound becomes incredibly problematic.

Dietary fatty acids play many roles in the body. One of their biggest functions is to be the metabolic building blocks for the body's production of a group of communication compounds called prostaglandins. Remember these? We met them in the last chapter. Essential fatty acids are incorporated into our cell membranes, and are a liberated by an enzyme called phospholipase, for use in daily metabolic processes - ie the formation of prostaglandins. Prostaglandins regulate several important responses in the body, including of course...the inflammatory response. There are 3 types of prostaglandin - series 1, series 2, and series 3. Series 1 is mildly anti-inflammatory, series 2 is powerfully pro-inflammatory (ie switches on and exacerbates inflammation), and series 3 is powerfully anti-inflammatory. Omega 6 when consumed at a level above our daily needs, gets converted into something called arachidonic acid. This can then be rapidly converted into series 2 prostaglandins - the powerfully pro-inflammatory variety. On average here in the UK, we are consuming 23 times more omega 6 than we need PER DAY!! The end result of this is that we are essentially force feeding metabolic pathways that manufacture prostaglandins, and our body's expression of the pro inflammatory series 2 goes into overdrive. It is pretty logical whats going to happen here. Then of course there are other omega 6 derived pro inflammatory eicosanoids.

A little bit good. Too much bad

Omega-6 fats are found in:

- Vegetable and seed oils (soybean, corn, sunflower, safflower, cottonseed)

- Processed foods (anything fried, packaged, or fast food)

- Conventional salad dressings, mayonnaise, and sauces

- Grain-fed meat and dairy (due to high omega-6 feed)

Traditionally, humans consumed omega-6 and omega-3 in a balanced 1:1 ratio, but today, the ratio is often 20:1 or higher, heavily skewed towards inflammatory omega-6 fats (Simopoulos, 2016). We need to get that back to a healthy ratio if we are to stand any chance of reducing inflammation.

On the flip side of all of this, we have the other big dietary fatty acid group & one you have probably heard a great deal about. Omega 3 fatty acids. These amazing fatty acids are literally like the antidote to the above. There are 3 main types of omega 3 fatty acid - ALA, EPA, and DHA. These are almost as good as a complete antidote to the above. As has been outlined, the essential fatty acids are the metabolic precursors to prostaglandins. EPA and DHA are actually metabolised to form series 3 prostaglandins (EPA more so). These are the ones that are the most potently anti-inflammatory, and an increase in their production can influence inflammatory events very quickly indeed. Consuming good quantities of Omega 3 fatty acids encourages our body to produce more of the anti-inflammatory prostaglandins. This will be covered in the next chapter.

Trans Fats: The Worst Fat for Inflammation

Now we will briefly move on to a completely different animal. An abominable beast that is man made and toxic. Trans fats (or partially hydrogenated oils) are artificial fats created when vegetable oils undergo hydrogenation—a process that turns liquid oil into a solid fat to extend shelf life. That is how something like margarine which is made out of vegetable oils that are usually liquid, and get it to become more solid and butter like. Hydrogen is bubbled through these oils and it causes their molecules to change. They flip around and become misshaped. Whilst yes this does make them a solid texture, it also makes them highly reactive and napalm for inflammation.

These fats are found in:

- Fast food (fried chicken, fries, nuggets, doughnuts)

- Margarine and vegetable shortening

- Processed baked goods (pastries, cookies, biscuits, cakes)

- Frozen processed foods (pizzas, pies, ready meals)

- Packaged snacks (crackers, chips, microwave popcorn)

Even though many governments have banned or limited trans fats, they can still be found in some processed foods under names like "partially hydrogenated oil."

Trans fats trigger inflammation in many ways. Firstly they *activate NF-κB*, that powerful inflammatory switch we met earlier that turns on the production of pro-inflammatory molecules (Mozaffarian et al., 2004).

Then we have the disruption of cell membranes. Cell membranes are made of fats, and their composition depends on the types of fats we eat. As I described earlier, fats and fatty acids are deposited into the cell membrane, and then released when they are needed. When trans fats replace healthy fats in cell membranes, they make cells more rigid which drastically impairs function.

The increased rigidity of the cell membranes when trans fats take a hold also leads to reduced cellular communication, affecting metabolism. Minerals have to cross membranes. Receptors for specific hormones and proteins are embedded within the membrane too. All of these are negatively affected.

Then finally we have disruption of the endothelium. This is the highly active inner skin that lines our blood vessels. It is vital for normal healthy functioning of the cardiovascular system, and any damage to the endothelium is what sets the wheels in motion for cardiovascular disease. Trans fats cause significant damage to this lining. This leads to arterial plaque formation (eventually), residual inflammation in the local area and poor vascular dynamics, leading to issues such as high blood pressure (Baer et al., 2004).

The simplest yet most powerful change that you can make to your diet when it comes to tackling inflammation is to change the type of fats that you are using in your diet and to increase your intake of others. That will be a key part of the plan.

Alcohol

The final dietary element to talk about is alcohol. This is always a contentious one and an area that I have become more mindful of as I get older. Many people enjoy a drink now and then—whether it's a glass of wine with dinner or a few beers on the weekend. But what if alcohol is quietly fuelling chronic inflammation inside your body, increasing the risk of disease? Well...it is!

While moderate alcohol intake has been linked to some potential health benefits, there's no escaping the fact that alcohol is a toxin. The feelings that it gives us are actually the body fighting that toxin. It disrupts immune function, damages the gut, and triggers systemic inflammation—all of which play a role in conditions like heart disease, autoimmune disorders, liver disease, and even mental health problems.

So, let's break it all down. How exactly does alcohol drive inflammation? What happens inside your body when you drink? And, most importantly, how can you protect yourself while still enjoying life?

How Alcohol Fuels Inflammation in the Body

Drinking alcohol triggers multiple inflammatory responses throughout the body. The effects depend on how much you drink, how often, and individual factors like genetics, gut health, and diet. Here's how alcohol contributes to chronic inflammation:

One of the first systems to take a pounding when we consume too much alcohol is the gut. Earlier in this book we covered how issues such as dysbiosis and break down of barrier function can create an inflammatory tidal wave. Well, alcohol is a huge driver of this.

Alcohol damages the tight junctions, those protein bands that keep our enterocytes (gut wall cells) tightly bound together.

This in turn leads to increased permeability of the gut, some-times called leaky gut syndrome. This, as we saw can cause toxins, bacteria, and undigested food particles leak into the bloodstream. This causes an immune response as something foreign has entered our circulation. This in turn then triggers an immune response, causing the release of *pro-inflammatory cytokines like IL-6 and TNF-a* (Bishehsari et al., 2017).

A breakdown in barrier function, where the gut gets 'leaky' allows *lipopolysaccharides (LPS)*—toxic molecules from gut bacteria—to enter the bloodstream, causing metabolic endo-toxemia and systemic inflammation (Wang et al., 2010). I wont go over that again as it is clearly described in the previous sec-tion of the book. Leaky gut also fuels autoimmune disorders, as the immune system starts attacking not just toxins, but also healthy tissues. Keeping this enclosed system healthy is vital.

Alcohol also damages the gut by having an impact upon the microbiome. It can soon disrupt the balance between bene-ficial and more harmful bacterial varieties. Remember, many of the beneficial bacteria within our microbiome regulate im-mune function and inflammation. Alcohol throws this delicate ecosystem out of balance, leading to dysbiosis (gut bacteria imbalance). Excessive alcohol consumption lowers the bene-ficial bacteria *(Lactobacillus, Bifidobacterium)*, which normally keep inflammation in check. This strain of bacteria is also a key player in digestive processes and in the regulation of the im-mediate environment of the gut such as assisting in the protec-tion against harmful dysbiotic bacteria. Alcohol also promotes the growth of inflammatory bacteria, increasing production of harmful compounds like LPS (Mutlu et al., 2009). With this al-teration in the microbiome, there is a reduction in the synthe-sis of short-chain fatty acids (SCFAs), which play a role in gut healing and immune regulation. It paints a pretty sorry picture for the gut.

Then of course we have the impact that alcohol has on the liver. Yes when there is excessive consumption over time, we know that it can physically change and damage the liver, but what about regular consumption at normal levels. Well, that can cause problems to when we are at the upper end of that. An overwhelmed or struggling liver can lead to:

- Fat buildup in liver cells (fatty liver disease). This increases the risk of insulin resistance and triggers a cascade of inflammatory events. If not improved over time this can lead to liver fibrosis and even eventually cirrhosis.

- Increased oxidative stress, which damages liver tissue (Szabo & Saha, 2015). That constant oxidative stress will accelerate scarring but also will continually fan the flames of inflammation which

- Production of inflammatory molecules, including TNF-α and IL-1β. We met these earlier on so you know the consequences of an elevation of these.

When the liver is overburdened, it releases inflammatory chemicals into the bloodstream, contributing to chronic inflammation and disease (Mandrekar & Szabo, 2009). The issue no longer just remains local. It gets things fired up systemically too.

There is a considerable effect upon our wider metabolic health too. Alcohol also notably interferes with blood sugar control, which plays a direct role in inflammation, not to mention weight gain, cardiovascular disease and type 2 diabetes risk. You will see throughout this book and as a key part of the plan that blood glucose regulation will become a focal point in the long term management of inflammation.

Alcohol causes blood sugar spikes and crashes, leading to an inflammatory response (Paresh et al., 2006). There are a lot of simple sugars in alcohol and also when we consume it, as a toxin its clearance takes priority in the body. Constituents from the food that we eat are not metabolised as rapidly as they would be. So, things like lipids and glucose in the blood hang around for longer whilst our body prioritises dealing with the toxic onslaught. This can cause further spikes in blood glucose. Put all the variables together and it can cause havoc with blood sugar.

Chronic drinking increases insulin resistance over time if this consistent blood sugar carpet bombing continues. If insulin resistance develops it can also raise inflammation markers like C-reactive protein (CRP).

Then, the final area that alcohol affects from an inflammatory point of view is the brain and the nervous system. Ever feel mentally foggy after drinking? That's because alcohol triggers inflammation in the brain. We spoke about neuroinflammation in the previous section, this is the same thing but with a much more acute onset. If you drink a lot regularly, this state will stick.

Alcohol activates microglia, the brain's immune cells, leading to neuroinflammation (Crews et al., 2017). Chronic drinking is linked to increased Alzheimer's and dementia risk (Matsui et al., 2017). It also reduces brain-derived neurotrophic factor (BDNF), a molecule essential for brain function and memory.

All in all, alcohol is something that we do need to consider keeping to a minimum. Not being the fun police here but if you seriously want to get to grips with inflammation and put yourself in the best possible position, then consider cutting back.

CHAPTER 6:
THE ANTI-INFLAMMATORY FOODS TO POWER YOUR PLATE

We know that aspects of our diet and lifestyle can drive chronic inflammation. But what are we supposed to do about it all? Thankfully there are a lot of foods we can include and tweaks and swaps that we can make in our daily diets that will have a significant impact. The beauty is too that these swaps and tweaks are very easy to make and the end result is not only better health. It is delicious food on our plates too. Let's get into it.

Increase The Omega 3. Cut The Omega 6

Of course we have to start here! That horror story I told you in the previous chapter should have you ditching sunflower oil like it is an unexploded bomb. The oils we consume, and more importantly the fatty acids that they contain have a dramatic impact upon inflammation in our body. One of the most powerful changes to your diet that you could possibly make, is to cut out the omega 6 rich oils, and increase your intake of long chain omega 3 fatty acids. I will go into more specific detail about what the omega 3's are in a moment but, these are anti-inflammatory power houses. As a rule we are not consuming anywhere near the amount of omega 3 fatty acids that we need. Especially the active long chain varieties, and this has a serious impact on our long term health in a multitude of ways.

There could be an entire book dedicated to just that. When it comes to inflammation, making that shift in the type of fatty acids that you are prioritising in your daily diet really can work miracles

You may well have come across the debate about omega-6 vs. omega-3 fatty acids. Certainly if you paid attention in the previous chapters you will be very familiar. Some say omega-6 fats are inflammatory, while others claim they're essential and nothing to worry about, or that any such claim about such oils is simply hogwash. The truth lies somewhere in between. We do absolutely need both omega-6 and omega-3 fats, but we need them in the right balance. Unfortunately, modern diets, because of the types of foods I mentioned previously, have completely tipped the scales in favour of omega-6, fuelling chronic inflammation and increasing the risk of long-term health issues.

For thousands of years, humans ate a diet where omega-6 and omega-3 fatty acids were fairly balanced, at about a 1:1 or 2:1 ratio. But today, thanks to processed foods, vegetable oils, and grain-fed animal products, the typical Western diet has an omega-6 to omega-3 ratio of 15:1 or even 20:1 (Simopoulos, 2016). Here in the UK it can get as far as 25:1. This shift is a massive problem for inflammation, because these two fats compete for the same enzymes and influence the body's production of inflammatory and anti-inflammatory compounds.

By increasing omega-3 intake while reducing omega-6 consumption, you can push your body back into balance, helping to lower inflammation, improve immune function, and support brain, heart, and metabolic health. Let's break down exactly how this works and why it's one of the most powerful dietary changes you can make.

The Omega-6 and Omega-3 Tug of War: How It Affects Inflammation

The way omega-6 and omega-3 fats impact inflammation comes down to their role in eicosanoid production. We met these substances earlier, but here's a recap. Eicosanoids are signalling molecules that control inflammation, blood clotting, and immune responses. Omega-6 fats (especially arachidonic acid, or AA) produce eicosanoids that promote inflammation, blood clotting, and immune activation, while omega-3 fats - particularly the long chain variants (EPA and DHA) that we find in foods such as oily fish, produce eicosanoids that reduce inflammation, support tissue repair, and help resolve immune responses (Calder, 2017).

When your diet is overloaded with omega-6 fats and lacking omega-3s, your body is constantly producing pro-inflammatory compounds, leading to chronic low-grade inflammation. This is the kind of inflammation that doesn't go away and contributes to problems like heart disease, arthritis, autoimmune conditions, and even cognitive decline that we are focusing on here in this book. This isn't the acute stuff that benefits us. This is that slow burner that pushes us into a disease state over time (Calder, 2017).

The reason that we produce more. Well, both omega 3 and omega 6 rely on the same enzymes to turn them into their eicosanoid end products. These enzymes morph them and change them to eventually turn these fatty acids into eicosanoids. Some that are pro inflammatory. Some that are anti inflammatory. It is a simple numbers game really. The more of one type of fatty acid, the more of its related eicosanoid group will be produced. There is simply more of the starting material so there will be more of the end product. Makes sense. A small amount of omega 6 goes down a very beneficial enzyme pathway and is converted into something called GLA which is very beneficial. However, this pathways gets full up with just the tiniest amount of omega 6. Once it is full, the excess omega 6 goes down the main enzyme pathway and gets converted into pro inflammatory eicosanoids that fan the inflammatory flame.

By increasing omega-3 intake, the omega 3 fatty acids compete with Omega 6 fatty acids for enzyme access, leading to a shift from inflammatory eicosanoids to more anti-inflammatory and inflammation-resolving compounds like resolvins, protectins, and maresins (Serhan & Chiang, 2013). These specialised molecules help turn off unnecessary inflammation, preventing it from lingering and causing long-term damage.

How Omega-3s Shut Down the Inflammatory Cascade

Beyond balancing out omega-6-driven inflammation, omega-3s actively suppress major inflammatory pathways. One of the key ways they do this is by blocking NF-κB, the master switch for inflammation. NF-κB controls the production of several inflammatory cytokines, including TNF-α, IL-6, and IL-1β, which drive chronic diseases like atherosclerosis, metabolic syndrome, and autoimmune disorders (Minihane et al., 2016).

Diets rich in omega-6 fats have been shown to activate NF-κB, leading to a steady increase in inflammatory cytokines. This is especially problematic for people dealing with conditions like rheumatoid arthritis, inflammatory bowel disease, and even depression, where chronic inflammation plays a major role (Calder, 2017).

On the other hand, when you increase omega-3 intake, especially EPA and DHA, these fats inhibit NF-κB, reducing the production of inflammatory cytokines and oxidative stress (Calder, 2017). Multiple studies have found that higher omega-3 intake leads to lower levels of CRP (C-reactive protein), TNF-α, and IL-6, all of which are markers of systemic inflammation (Minihane et al., 2016).

For example, in patients with rheumatoid arthritis, supplementing with omega-3s has been shown to reduce joint pain, stiffness, and swelling, even allowing some individuals to lower their reliance on anti-inflammatory medications (Calder, 2017). Similarly, in people with heart disease, omega-3s help lower vascular inflammation, improving blood vessel function and reducing the risk of cardiovascular events (Mozaffarian & Wu, 2012). There is a whole section dedicated to supplements in this book, so I will expand on that a lot more there.

Omega-3s, Immunity, and Autoimmune Diseases

One of the lesser-known but crucial roles of omega-3s is their effect on immune system regulation. Chronic inflammation isn't just about an overproduction of inflammatory molecules—it's also about an overactive, dysregulated immune system. This is particularly important in autoimmune diseases, where the immune system mistakenly attacks the body's own tissues.

Omega-3 fatty acids help restore immune balance by increasing the activity of regulatory T cells (Tregs), which prevent the immune system from overreacting (Calder, 2017). At the same time, they reduce the activity of M1 macrophages, which are the pro-inflammatory immune cells responsible for excessive immune activation. Instead, they promote the M2 macrophage phenotype, which calms inflammation and supports tissue repair (Serhan & Chiang, 2013).

This is why omega-3 intake has been shown to be beneficial for conditions like multiple sclerosis, lupus, psoriasis, and ulcerative colitis. Studies have found that people with higher omega-3 intake experience fewer flare-ups, reduced symptom severity, and better overall disease management (Simopoulos, 2016).

Brain Inflammation and Mental Health: The Role of DHA

As we saw earlier, something that surprises most people is the fact that many of the mental health and neurodegeneratve conditions that are plaguing us, actually involve an inflammatory element. Neuroinflammation. It is a known factor in conditions like depression, anxiety, Alzheimer's disease, and cognitive decline (Bazan, 2018).

DHA, the most abundant omega-3 in the brain, helps regulate inflammation by reducing the activation of microglia, the brain's immune cells. When microglia are chronically activated, they produce pro-inflammatory cytokines that contribute to neurodegeneration and mental health disorders (Bazan, 2018).

Research has found that people with depression often have lower levels of DHA and higher levels of pro-inflammatory cytokines, suggesting that neuroinflammation plays a major role in mood disorders (Mocking et al., 2016). Studies have shown that increasing omega-3 intake, particularly DHA, can significantly reduce depressive symptoms, especially in individuals with high levels of inflammation (Mocking et al., 2016).

This is why omega-3-rich foods and supplements are increasingly being recommended not just for brain health, but also for mood support and mental resilience.

It Is The Form That Counts

So, that was a lot to take in I know. But....there's more. It isn't as simple as just knocking back any form of omega 3 and assuming it will do you good. Omega 3 is not one single substance. Omega-3 fatty acids come in several forms, but the most powerful and bioavailable types are the long-chain omega-3s—eicosapentaenoic acid (EPA) and docosahexaenoic acid (DHA). These fats are found predominantly in marine sources like fatty fish and algae, and they are the key players when it comes to lowering inflammation, supporting brain health, and improving cardiovascular function.

There is another form of omega-3, alpha-linolenic acid (ALA), which is found in plant-based sources like flaxseeds, chia seeds, and walnuts. While ALA is still an essential fatty acid and offers some minimal health benefits, humans convert ALA into EPA and DHA very inefficiently. This is a major reason why direct consumption of EPA and DHA from fish or supplements is far more effective at reducing inflammation than relying on plant-based omega-3 sources alone. Here's why.

Omega-3 fatty acids are categorised based on their chain length—the number of carbon atoms in their structure. Long-chain omega-3s (EPA and DHA) contain 20 or more carbon atoms, while short-chain omega-3s (ALA) contain only 18 carbon atoms.

The longer carbon chains of EPA and DHA make them structurally and functionally superior to ALA. These fats integrate more efficiently into cell membranes, particularly in the brain, heart, and immune cells, where they exert their powerful anti-inflammatory effects (Calder, 2017). They are also put straight into action.

EPA plays a crucial role in reducing inflammation, while DHA is highly concentrated in the brain and nervous system, where it is essential for cognitive function, neuroprotection, and mental health. Both EPA and DHA contribute to the production of resolvins and protectins, which actively help resolve inflammation and promote tissue healing (Serhan & Chiang, 2013). These two long chain omega 3 fatty acids are put straight into their key areas of use as soon as we consume them.

In contrast, ALA must first be converted into EPA and DHA before the body can utilise it for these functions. It goes through a series of enzymes in order to be lengthened and stretched and eventually be turned into the highly active long chain varieties. Unfortunately, humans are extremely poor at making this conversion, which means relying on plant-based omega-3 sources may not provide adequate amounts of the most beneficial forms. In fact I can guarantee it.

On average, the conversion rate of ALA to EPA is less than 10%, and the conversion to DHA is even worse—typically less than 1% (Brenna et al., 2009). This means that even if someone consumes a high amount of ALA from plant sources like flaxseeds or walnuts, they are still unlikely to produce enough EPA and DHA to experience the full anti-inflammatory benefits.

The conversion of ALA into long-chain omega-3s as we have seen is dependent on a series of enzyme-driven steps, involving delta-6 desaturase and delta-5 desaturase enzymes. These enzymes are also used in the metabolism of omega-6 fatty acids. Since most modern diets are overloaded with omega-6 fats, these enzymes are often already occupied converting omega-6 fats into pro-inflammatory arachidonic acid (AA), leaving even fewer resources available to convert ALA into EPA and DHA (Brenna et al., 2009).

Other factors that further reduce the conversion efficiency of ALA include:

- Genetics – Some people naturally have lower conversion rates due to genetic variations.

- Age – Conversion rates decline with age, making it even harder for older individuals to produce sufficient EPA and DHA from ALA.

- Sex – Women tend to convert ALA into EPA and DHA slightly better than men, but the conversion is still poor overall.

- Nutrient Deficiencies – The conversion process requires zinc, magnesium, and B vitamins, which are commonly low in Western diets.

This inefficient conversion is why relying on flaxseeds, chia seeds, walnuts, and other plant-based sources of ALA is not enough to provide optimal levels of EPA and DHA. While these foods are still healthy and provide beneficial fiber, lignans, and antioxidants, they should not be considered a primary source of omega-3s for inflammation control.

Since EPA and DHA are the directly active forms of omega-3s, they bypass the inefficient conversion process required by ALA and get to work immediately in the body. They should be the priority in our quest to increase our omega 3 intake.

Although, one little note here. ALA can influence inflammation in a mild way and can contribute to the overall picture. This is because, even though it is not well converted into EPA & DHA, it still occupies the same enzymes that omega 6 would try and occupy. Even if the end product, ie the long chain omega 3's does not really happen, ALA will still be preventing some omega 6 from occupying those enzymes and as such will prevent some from being turned into the pro inflammatory eicosanoids that are associated with omega 6. So, plant sources of omega 3 do contribute to the overall picture because they prevent some omega 6 causing problems.

This is why you will see me use ingredients such as flax seeds, walnuts, flax oil etc just to help us tip things in our favour.

How to get a better balance for life

Balancing your omega-3 and omega-6 intake isn't just about adding more omega-3s—it's also about reducing excess omega-6 intake. This means:

- Cutting back on processed vegetable oils like soybean, corn, sunflower, and safflower oil.

- Avoiding fried and ultra-processed foods, which are loaded with omega-6-rich oils.

- Choosing grass-fed meats, pasture-raised eggs, and wild-caught fish instead of grain-fed animal products.

- Eating more fatty fish (salmon, sardines, mackerel, anchovies) for a direct source of EPA and DHA.

- Considering the right kinds of supplements.

Opt For High Fibre Slow Burning Carbohydrates

The next thing that is going to benefit you drastically, and that is a fundamental part to this plan, is making the right carbohydrate choice. Carbohydrates are a key component of the human diet, providing the primary source of energy for our cells, fuelling everything from brain function to muscle activity. We need to have some in our diet. However as we have seen, not all carbohydrates are created equal, particularly when it comes to their impact on inflammation. The modern diet is heavily saturated with refined carbohydrates—highly processed, stripped of fibre and essential nutrients—resulting in metabolic chaos that fuels chronic inflammation. These foods, including white bread, pasta, pastries, and sugar-laden beverages, cause rapid spikes in blood sugar and insulin levels, leading to metabolic dysfunction, fat accumulation, and the activation of inflammatory pathways. These are the ones that we are going to be ditching. For good! Plus as a rule we eat far more carbohydrates than we actually need, so we will be becoming much more mindful of carbohydrate portions as we go along.

Refined carbohydrates—such as white bread, white rice, pastries, and sugar-sweetened products—are digested rapidly which releases all of their glucose in one short hit, causing sharp spikes in blood glucose and insulin levels. This sudden surge in sugar triggers a cascade of inflammatory processes in the body, leading to increased production of inflammatory cytokines, oxidative stress, and long-term metabolic dysfunction (Esposito et al., 2002).

By contrast, high-fibre, low-glycemic carbohydrates such as non-starchy vegetables, legumes, nuts, seeds, and minimally processed whole grains act in the opposite way. They slow digestion, promote blood sugar stability, enhance gut health, and reduce inflammatory markers throughout the body. The high fibre content means that their glucose is liberated far more slowly which drip feeds blood sugar, keeping it even and stable. Making the switch from refined carbohydrates to these slow-digesting, nutrient-rich alternatives is one of the most powerful dietary strategies to combat chronic inflammation and prevent disease. Making this shift offers profound anti-inflammatory benefits, primarily by improving blood sugar control, supporting gut health, and reducing insulin resistance.

Then we have the added benefit that choosing this type of carbohydrate source, and the amount of fibre contained within them has a hugely beneficial effect upon the gut, and addresses many of the things we addressed earlier in relation to reduced barrier function and increased intestinal permeability risk. The gut microbiome—the trillions of bacteria residing in the digestive tract—plays a critical role in immune function and inflammatory regulation. When properly balanced, the microbiome produces beneficial short-chain fatty acids (SCFAs) such as butyrate, acetate, and propionate, which lower inflammation, strengthen the gut barrier, and modulate immune responses (Rooks & Garrett, 2016). How to we create a better balance and increase the production of these short chain fatty acids? We eat fibre. Within these high fibre foods are carbohydrates that do not get broken down by the pancreatic enzymes released in the small intestine in the same way that more simple carbohydrates do. Instead they are reliant on gut bacteria fermenting them don in a process called saccharolytic fermentation. Short chain fatty acids are a by product of this process.

Refined carbohydrates, devoid of fibre, feed pro-inflammatory bacteria, contributing to gut dysbiosis, increased intestinal permeability (leaky gut), and systemic inflammation. By contrast, fibre-rich carbohydrates encourage the growth of beneficial bacteria, leading to increased SCFA production. SCFAs directly reduce NF-κB activation, lower inflammatory cytokine production, and improve gut barrier integrity, preventing harmful molecules from entering the bloodstream (Cani et al., 2007). Get them down you!

By incorporating more low-glycemic carbohydrate sources— such as non-starchy vegetables, berries, legumes, nuts, and whole grains in moderation—blood sugar fluctuations are minimised, microbiome diversity is ensured, gut health improves dramatically, and inflammation levels decline.

Best High-Fibre Low-Glycemic Carbohydrates To Use Frequently

Category	Food Item	Fibre Content (Per 100g)	Glycemic Index (GI)	Health Benefits
Grains	Oats (Rolled or Steel-Cut)	10g	55 (Medium)	Rich in beta-glucans, supports heart health and blood sugar control.
Grains	Barley	17g	25 (Low)	High in soluble fibre, aids digestion and cholesterol reduction.
Grains	Quinoa	2.8g	53 (Medium)	Complete protein source, rich in essential amino acids.
Grains	Buckwheat	10g	50 (Low)	Gluten-free alternative, high in antioxidants.
Grains	Brown Basmati Rice	2.2g	55 (Medium)	Better glycemic control than white rice, provides sustained energy.
Grains	Rye Berries	15g	34 (Low)	Good source of iron and magnesium, supports gut health.

Legumes	Lentils	8g	32 (Low)	High in protein and iron, supports muscle and blood health.
Legumes	Chickpeas	7.6g	28 (Low)	Rich in folate and fibre, beneficial for gut microbiota.
Legumes	Black Beans	8.7g	30 (Low)	Supports gut health, high in antioxidants.
Legumes	Butter Beans	7.1g	36 (Low)	Creamy texture, rich in potassium and fibre.
Legumes	Red Kidney Beans	6.4g	24 (Low)	Lowers cholesterol and improves blood sugar regulation.
Legumes	Garden Peas	5.1g	48 (Medium)	Supports digestion, rich in plant-based protein.
Starchy Vegetables	Sweet Potatoes	3g	50 (Medium)	Rich in beta-carotene, supports vision and immune function.
Starchy Vegetables	Butternut Squash	2g	51 (Medium)	Good source of vitamin A, supports healthy skin.
Starchy Vegetables	Carrots	2.8g	39 (Low)	High in carotenoids and fibre, supports digestive health.
Starchy Vegetables	Parsnips	4.9g	52 (Medium)	Provides natural sweetness, supports gut motility.

That should give you a bit of an idea for the kind of carbohydrate choices you should be making. In practice it really is very simple. The biggest step is to ditch the white refined stuff and opt for the high fibre slow burners.

Another key component here though, to really amplify these blood sugar regulating effects, is what you consume the carbohydrate sources with. The first part of the picture is indeed opting for these types of high fibre slow burning carbs. The next consideration is how the meal is assembled. Just because these types of carbohydrates are slow burners, it doesn't mean that you will just chow down on a great big bowl full of wholewheat pasta. That will still send blood glucose levels through the roof and fan the inflammatory flame. We need to ensure that our meals are balanced. You can get too much of a good thing.

Where possible, at each meal we need to make sure that the plate is balanced. What do I mean by balanced? Well, on each plate ensure there is - a serving of these slow burning high fibre carbohydrates. A portion of a high quality protein, some healthy fats and as many brightly coloured non starchy as you want. Think a baked salmon fillet with some brown rice and stir fried greens. Or a chicken breast, baked potato and roasted peppers. It doesn't need to be complicated, just balanced.

Why do I recommend this? Protein and healthy fats will dramatically slow down the digestion of meals. This slowing of digestion not only helps to keep you full and prevent hunger pangs, but it also means that the glucose content of the meal will be liberated even more slowly, ensuring the gradual drip feeding of our blood sugar and keeping the aggressive inflammatory responses to elevated glucose at bay. When you add these foods to carbohydrate sources that are already of a low glycemic value and that are high in fibre and slow burners and slow to digest, you create a meal that will just gently drip feed your blood sugar instead of carpet bombing it. This gradual drip feeding of blood glucose will help to prevent blood sugar and insulin spikes that pour petrol on the flames of inflamma-tion.

The diagram below will show you how to balance your plates. if you look for this kind of visual meal combination, using the right ingredients in the right proportions, then you really will be on the right track for your day to day eating.

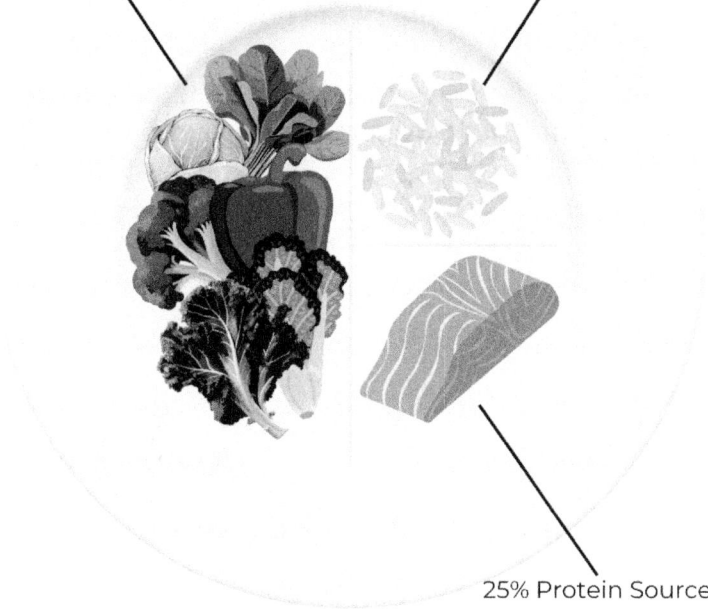

50% Non Starchy Veg

25% High Fibre, Slow Burning Carbohydrate

25% Protein Source

Pile Up The Anti-Inflammatory, Phytochemical-Rich Foods

The next thing that we are going to be adding in abundance are foods rich in bioactive compounds such as polyphenols, flavonols, flavonoids and all of these great things that sound hellishly complicated but really are just powerful plant chemicals that amongst other things have a known and recorded anti-inflammatory activity. These tend to be the brightly coloured fruits and vegetables and it tends to be the chemistry that gives them their bright colours that also delivers their benefits too. Brightly coloured fruits and vegetables have long been celebrated for their potential to combat inflammation. From the deep purple of blackberries to the vivid orange of carrots, these foods are often brimming with phytonutrients that can modulate inflammatory processes in the body. The precise mechanisms vary, yet many share a few core strategies: quenching free radicals, down regulating pro-inflammatory cytokines, and supporting beneficial gut microbes. What follows is an exploration of several common fruits and vegetables noted for their anti-inflammatory activity. While their flavours and appearances may differ widely, each contributes, in its own way, to dialling back the chronic, low-grade inflammation that underlies numerous modern health concerns.

Fruit:

Apples

We all know what an apple a day doesApples, though often seen as a dependable, everyday fruit, are by no means lacking in anti-inflammatory clout. Their skins contain an array of flavonoids, including quercetin, which is notable for its antioxidant and anti-inflammatory attributes (Hyson, 2011). Quercetin can inhibit the release of histamine and other mediators involved in both allergy and inflammation (Middleton et al., 2000). In addition, apples include pectin, a soluble fiber that fosters a healthy gut microbiome. A balanced microbiome exerts a powerful influence on inflammatory processes throughout the body, partly by reinforcing the integrity of the intestinal barrier, thereby preventing unwelcome substances from escaping into the bloodstream and perpetuating systemic inflammation (Bischoff, 2011). As is often suggested, consuming apples with their peel ensures a higher intake of both fiber and phytonutri-ents—provided, of course, that they are washed thoroughly or sourced organically.

Blackberries

Blackberries, with their dark hue and slightly tart sweetness, have attracted research attention due to their high content of anthocyanins. These pigments give blackberries their distinctive color and possess significant antioxidant properties (Wu et al., 2004). Antioxidants help neutralize free radicals—unstable molecules that can damage cells and incite inflammatory responses. When free radicals accumulate, they often trigger the release of cytokines like TNF-α and interleukin-6 (IL-6), which perpetuate a cycle of inflammation (Aggarwal and Shishodia, 2006). By scavenging these harmful species, blackberries ease oxidative stress before it morphs into chronic inflammation. Studies also suggest that polyphenols in blackberries may inhibit the activity of nuclear factor kappa B (NF-κB), a transcription factor that governs the expression of various pro-inflammatory genes (Nile and Park, 2014). While one serving of blackberries is not a magic bullet, regularly incorporating them into the diet can steadily help lower the inflammatory load.

Blueberries

Similar to blackberries, blueberries boast deep bluish-purple pigments linked to anthocyanins. In fact, blueberries are often touted as one of the richest dietary sources of these compounds, which have been studied for myriad potential health benefits, including cardioprotective and anti-inflammatory effects (Kalt et al., 2020). Research on adults with metabolic syndrome suggests that daily blueberry consumption may reduce oxidative stress markers and inflammatory cytokines, hinting at broader implications for conditions like hypertension and insulin resistance (Basu et al., 2010). Another avenue through which blueberries may ease inflammation is by enhancing endothelial function. When blood vessels are healthy and flexible, inflammatory processes involved in cardiovascular disease have less opportunity to take hold (Rodriguez-Mateos et al., 2013). One appealing feature of blueberries is that their anthocyanins remain relatively stable when frozen, so even off-season, frozen blueberries can deliver meaningful anti-inflammatory potential.

Cherries

Cherries, especially tart varieties like Montmorency cherries, have garnered attention for their capacity to alleviate inflammation and pain associated with conditions such as gout and osteoarthritis (Bell et al., 2014). The key players are anthocyanins and various phenolic acids, which help repress enzymes involved in generating inflammatory compounds. Similar to raspberries, cherries can reduce COX-2 activity, thereby diminishing the production of prostaglandins (Zafra-Stone et al., 2007). Research has also documented improvements in sleep quality tied to cherry consumption, partly attributed to melatonin content. While melatonin is more typically associated with regulating circadian rhythms, it also possesses antioxidant properties that combat oxidative stress (Burkhardt et al., 2001). The combined effect may offer wide-ranging support, from reducing inflammatory triggers to bolstering overall recovery, making cherries a useful addition for those interested in a comprehensive approach to health.

Grapefruit

Who remembers the grapefruit diet? Old school. Well, these sour fruits are incredibly good for you. Grapefruit is rich in naringenin, a flavonoid that inhibits Toll-like receptor (TLR) signalling, a key pathway in chronic inflammation (Jia et al., 2020). Naringenin also reduces lipid peroxidation, mitigating oxidative stress-induced inflammation (Borges et al., 2018). Moreover, grapefruit consumption has been linked to improved metabolic health by modulating adipokine expression and reducing insulin resistance (Ghanim et al., 2011).

Lemons and Limes

These do more than just stop sailors getting scurvy! Lemons and limes are abundant in vitamin C and flavonoids such as eriocitrin and hesperidin, which exhibit anti-inflammatory effects. These compounds scavenge reactive oxygen species (ROS) and inhibit NF-κB activation, reducing inflammatory cytokine production (Lima et al., 2019). Additionally, citrus flavonoids have been shown to enhance lipid metabolism and reduce obesity-associated inflammation (Peluso et al., 2018).

Oranges

Oranges contain high levels of hesperidin, a flavanone with well-documented anti-inflammatory properties. Hesperidin modulates mitogen-activated protein kinase (MAPK) signalling, reducing the expression of inflammatory cytokines (Grosso et al., 2017). Additionally, orange polyphenols improve vascular health by enhancing nitric oxide synthesis and reducing endothelial dysfunction (Guo et al., 2020).

Pomegranate

I always struggled with these as a kid, but these days I do love the juice and find that it makes an excellent base for smoothie concoctions. Pomegranates are rich in punicalagins and ellagic acid, pomegranates have been studied for their robust antioxidant capacity (Gil et al., 2000). These unique polyphenols can protect LDL cholesterol from oxidation, a process known to spark inflammatory changes in arterial walls that lead to atherosclerosis (Aviram and Dornfeld, 2001). By preventing LDL from becoming an irritant, pomegranates indirectly tamp down vascular inflammation. Human trials investigating pomegranate juice consumption have shown reductions in inflammatory biomarkers, along with improvements in blood pressure and cholesterol parameters (Rozenberg et al., 2006). The synergy among pomegranate's various polyphenols is a likely explanation for these broad-spectrum effects; single isolates rarely replicate the full impact of the whole fruit. Whether enjoyed as fresh seeds (arils) or pressed into juice, pomegranate's vibrant hue and refreshing taste add both flavor and function to any anti-inflammatory plan.

Raspberries

Raspberries, whether red or the less common golden variety, also offer an impressive repertoire of antioxidants. Like blackberries, their anti-inflammatory effects hinge on abundant polyphenols, including ellagitannins and anthocyanins (Häkkinen and Törrönen, 2000). These compounds not only help quell free-radical-induced damage but may also influence signaling pathways in immune cells. For instance, certain raspberry phytochemicals appear to downregulate cyclooxygenase-2 (COX-2), an enzyme crucial for producing pro-inflammatory mediators known as prostaglandins (Zafra-Stone et al., 2007). Prostaglandins are often beneficial in acute responses—like healing a wound—but in excess, they can lead to ongoing pain and inflammation. By modulating COX-2, raspberries help maintain a healthier equilibrium. Their relatively high fiber content further supports metabolic health, curbing the blood sugar spikes that contribute to chronic inflammation (Esposito et al., 2002).

Plums

Plums, which transform into prunes when dried, bring to the table (and the digestive system) significant antioxidant activity anchored by phenolic compounds such as neochlorogenic and chlorogenic acids (Nakatani et al., 2000). These acids help offset oxidative stress and may reduce lipid peroxidation, a process that leads to damaged lipids which can trigger inflammatory responses in the arteries and other tissues. The fiber in plums also encourages healthy bowel function and fosters beneficial gut flora, both of which can modulate low-level inflammation arising from dysbiosis (Schmidt et al., 2014). Some studies in older adults hint that incorporating prunes may benefit bone health, another area where inflammatory processes often wreak havoc if left unchecked (Franklin et al., 2006). While plums tend to be an underutilized fruit in some regions, their sweet-tart flavor and functional attributes make them a valuable asset in any anti-inflammatory dietary portfolio.

Red Grapes

Red grapes provide another glimpse into how nature packages potent anti-inflammatory agents in appealing forms. Their skins are rich in resveratrol, a stilbene that has garnered a reputation for supporting cardiovascular function and exerting anti-inflammatory and antioxidant effects (Baur and Sinclair, 2006). Resveratrol appears to modulate the same NF-κB pathway targeted by anthocyanins and other polyphenols, albeit through slightly different molecular steps (Aggarwal and Shishodia, 2006). This synergy highlights a recurring theme among pigmented fruits: they converge on similar inflammation-related signaling pathways, multiplying the likelihood of a meaningful impact when consumed regularly. Red grapes can also provide smaller amounts of quercetin and other flavonols, further broadening their benefits. While wine made from red grapes does supply resveratrol, fresh grapes maintain the advantage of delivering fiber and avoiding the negative impacts that come with alcohol consumption when taken in excess.

Strawberries

Who doesn't love these? Strawberries share comparable anti-inflammatory credentials. Their bright red color is attributed to anthocyanins such as pelargonidin, which exerts antioxidant effects that can shield tissues from oxidative stress (Giampieri et al., 2012). Research has linked regular strawberry consumption with lower levels of C-reactive protein (CRP), a key inflammatory marker, in adults with risk factors for cardiovascular disease (Basu et al., 2010). Additionally, strawberries contain vitamin C and an assortment of polyphenols that fortify the body's endogenous antioxidant defenses, limiting the initial triggers of inflammation. Some investigations even suggest that strawberry extracts can modulate the activity of NF-κB in cellular models, potentially halting the production of inflammatory cytokines at their source (Hannum, 2004). Their easy availability and sweet, accessible flavor make strawberries an especially user-friendly choice for individuals aiming to incorporate more anti-inflammatory foods.. Finally, some good news about a food we actually love.

Vegetables:

Beetroot

Beetroot, with its striking crimson hue derived from pigments called betalains, has also demonstrated anti-inflammatory properties. Betalains are potent antioxidants that appear to inhibit the activity of enzymes such as COX-2 (Clifford et al., 2015). Clinical trials with beetroot juice have shown improvements in vascular function, blood pressure, and oxidative stress markers in individuals with hypertension or other cardiovascular risks, underscoring the synergy between anti-inflammatory and cardioprotective effects (Hobbs et al., 2012). Beetroot is also a source of dietary nitrates, which the body converts into nitric oxide (NO). NO not only supports healthy vasodilation, thereby lowering blood pressure, but may further influence inflammatory signaling pathways (Lundberg et al., 2008). Though some might find beets earthy or overpowering, roasting them to caramelize natural sugars or blending them into smoothies can make their flavor more appealing, all while delivering a punch of phytonutrient goodness.

Carrots

Carrots, known for their beta-carotene content, round out this list of colorful foods with anti-inflammatory potential. Beta-carotene is a precursor to vitamin A, important for immune function and cellular differentiation. Like other carotenoids, beta-carotene also exhibits antioxidant activity, limiting the formation of reactive oxygen species (Tanumihardjo, 2013). This means fewer triggers for chronic inflammatory pathways. Meanwhile, carrots also offer additional phytonutrients, such as luteolin, that can temper overactive immune responses. Research on luteolin suggests it may attenuate NF-κB signaling, thus lessening the production of inflammatory mediators (Seelinger et al., 2008). While carrots are often relegated to a simple side dish or raw snack, more creative approaches—like roasting them with herbs or blending them into soups—can maximize nutrient retention and enhance their appeal. Additionally, cooking can help break down the tough cell walls, making beta-carotene more bioavailable, similar to the lycopene effect in tomatoes.

Purple Sweet Potatoes

Hands down one of my favourite foods on earth! Purple sweet potatoes, while less common in some parts of the world, are particularly rich in anthocyanins—similar to berries—making them visually vibrant and nutritionally compelling (Teow et al., 2007). The antioxidant potency of these tubers helps mitigate lipid peroxidation and reduce oxidative stress, which, if unchecked, can trigger prolonged inflammatory states. Some research indicates that extracts from purple sweet potatoes may also modulate immune responses, reducing pro-inflammatory cytokine release in experimental models (Mohanraj and Sivasankar, 2014). They carry a blend of complex carbohydrates, fiber, and micronutrients (including vitamin A precursors) that collectively support metabolic health. Since inflammation often intersects with metabolic dysfunction, consistent consumption of nutrient-dense carbohydrates like purple sweet potatoes can offer broad, cumulative benefits.

Red Cabbage

Red cabbage provides a noteworthy vegetable alternative for those wanting anthocyanins outside of the berry realm. These anthocyanins, once again, serve as potent antioxidants and may inhibit key inflammatory enzymes. Their presence gives red cabbage its striking purplish hue, which can be particularly pronounced when the cabbage is consumed raw or lightly cooked (Wu et al., 2004). Similar to other cruciferous vegetables, red cabbage also offers glucosinolates, compounds that have shown promise in reducing oxidative stress and offering protection against certain forms of cancer (Traka and Mithen, 2009). Adding raw red cabbage to salads or lightly steaming it preserves many of these compounds, providing a fiber-rich, anti-inflammatory choice that also pairs well with a broad range of cuisines.

Red Onions

There is a very good reason why every savoury recipe that I make always starts off with these powerful purple flavour bombs. Red onions illustrate that it is not solely fruits that supply quercetin and anthocyanins. Their outer layers have some of the highest concentrations of quercetin among commonly eaten vegetables (Lachman et al., 2020). Quercetin can downregulate the production of pro-inflammatory mediators and protect cells from oxidative damage. It has also been linked to potential vascular benefits, such as improved endothelial function, which can help keep systemic inflammation under better control (Kelly, 2011). Red onions, being more sweet and mild than yellow onions, are often eaten raw, thereby retaining more of their quercetin content. Cooking can cause some phytonutrient loss, but moderate heat treatments typically only reduce—not eliminate—the onion's benefits. This means that whether thrown into a stir-fry, roasted with other vegetables, or sliced onto salads, red onions can contribute to a more balanced inflammatory milieu.

Tomatoes

Ok ok...I know...they are a fruit! But I am putting them in here. Ok? Tomatoes, famed for their high lycopene content, are another staple frequently spotlighted for anti-inflammatory benefits. Lycopene is a carotenoid that gives tomatoes their deep red color, and it thrives under heat. This means cooked or stewed tomatoes can sometimes deliver more bioavailable lycopene than raw ones (Shi and Le Maguer, 2000). Lycopene's antioxidant capacity helps defend cells from oxidative insults, and some work suggests it may reduce expression of pro-inflammatory cytokines and adhesion molecules implicated in atherosclerosis (Gerster, 1997). Beyond lycopene, tomatoes provide a range of vitamins and minerals (vitamin C, potassium) that can further support immune resilience. People sensitive to nightshades may want to monitor their tomato intake, but generally, tomatoes are widely recognized as beneficial components of anti-inflammatory or heart-healthy diets.

As you will see in the recipes that follow, these ingredients will come up often. I am not saying that these are magic bullets and as powerful as adjusting your fatty acid intake or sorting out the glycemic impact of your diet. But, when consumed regularly as an every day part of your diet, the compounds that they contain will start to have a cumulative effect on inflammatory load. As we put it all together, its effects will mount up. There is however another culinary powerhouse that we have to cover before we put this all into action...

Spice it up

Ok we have the fundamental diet framework laid out now. You know what fats to increase and what fats to avoid. You know that you need to opt for an overall low glycemic diet. You know that there are powerful, colourful everyday foods that can give you added extra anti inflammatory support. So, the final thing to do, is get a bit spicy!

Spices are some of the most powerful, most phytochemical rich edible plants that we have available. As a Medical Herbalist, spices make up a huge proportion of the materia medica that I would call upon when making herbal prescriptions. They are powerful. Like fruit and veg and their colours, many of the actions of spices are related to their distinct flavours. Of course there are hundreds of spices out there, but I want to cover those that are the most common and of course, the most powerful. Let's get into it.

The Power Houses

Turmeric

Turmeric (*Curcuma longa*) is probably the most instantly recognisable of the three, largely thanks to its vibrant golden hue, which lights up curries, soups, and teas. Behind that deep color lies curcumin, the most studied bioactive compound in turmeric. Curcumin is part of a family of compounds called curcuminoids, all of which demonstrate physiological activity, although curcumin is the star performer when it comes to inflammation (Hewlings and Kalman, 2017).

In simple terms, chronic inflammation is often propelled by an array of molecules that signal the immune system to remain on high alert. Turmeric's capacity to help mediate this process has a lot to do with its effect on nuclear factor kappa B (NF-κB), a transcription factor that directly or indirectly influences the production of several pro-inflammatory cytokines, including TNF-α (tumour necrosis factor alpha) and IL-6 (interleukin-6). By modulating the activity of NF-κB, curcumin helps ensure that these inflammatory signals do not spiral out of control (Aggarwal and Shishodia, 2006).

Another key to turmeric's impact on inflammation lies in how it affects enzymes like cyclooxygenase-2 (COX-2) and lipoxygenase (LOX). These enzymes are involved in producing prostaglandins and leukotrienes, respectively—substances that can exacerbate inflammation if generated in excess (Menon and Sudheer, 2007). When curcumin gently reigns in the activity of COX-2 and LOX, it interrupts the cascade of chemical messengers that otherwise keep inflammatory pathways fuelled. On top of these biochemical interactions, turmeric exhibits robust antioxidant properties that mop up free radicals, thus defusing a major contributor to ongoing low-level inflammation (Sharma et al., 2005).

Human studies lend weight to these laboratory findings. Several randomised controlled trials have explored the use of curcumin supplements in conditions like osteoarthritis and rheumatoid arthritis, both of which feature prominent inflammatory components. Results often show decreases in joint pain and stiffness alongside measurable reductions in inflammatory markers (Kunnumakkara et al., 2016). Although not a universal remedy, turmeric's reliable presence in many therapeutic regimens highlights its potential to serve as an adjunct alongside other interventions.

Still, one important caveat is that curcumin has limited bioavailability when consumed alone. The body breaks it down swiftly in the liver and intestinal walls, which can curb the amount that actually makes it into systemic circulation (Shoba et al., 1998). This is why turmeric is often paired with black pepper—piperine from black pepper slows the breakdown of curcumin, thereby boosting the bioavailability. Including a source of dietary fat, such as coconut milk or olive oil, can also help enhance curcumin absorption since it is fat-soluble. Notably, people from traditional culinary cultures that have long used turmeric typically prepare it in fat-based sauces or stews, unknowingly facilitating the absorption of curcumin long before scientists had teased out the mechanisms.

In addition to its anti-inflammatory prowess, turmeric can influence metabolic health markers, many of which tie back to inflammation. Chronic inflammation often accompanies elevated blood glucose levels, dyslipidemia, or insulin resistance. Curcumin appears capable of improving insulin sensitivity by targeting inflammatory pathways that intersect with metabolic processes (Na et al., 2011). This coupling between inflammation and metabolism underlines turmeric's broad relevance; in many cases, addressing low-grade inflammation helps the body better manage blood glucose and lipid profiles, and turmeric emerges as a valuable culinary ally in that effort.

Of course, it's best to view turmeric as part of a broader dietary framework rather than a panacea. Adding more turmeric to meals, or occasionally supplementing with standardised extracts, can contribute to an anti-inflammatory lifestyle but works best in harmony with other nutrient-rich whole foods, sufficient protein intake, regular physical activity, and stress management. The synergy between these elements amplifies turmeric's protective, balancing effect on inflammation, and ensures that the rest of one's lifestyle also supports its benefits.

Garlic

Garlic (*Allium sativum*) has a pungent aroma that has often been described as both irresistible in the kitchen and daunting on the breath. Yet behind those robust sulphurous compounds lies an equally robust tradition of medicinal use that stretches across numerous cultures. For centuries, garlic has been valued not only for its flavour but also for its reputed ability to fend off infections, boost cardiovascular health, and support immune function (Rivlin, 2001). Modern studies highlight that many of these effects tie back to garlic's influence on inflammation.

Allicin, one of garlic's main bioactive compounds, is formed when garlic cloves are crushed or chopped. It is part of a broader family of sulfur-containing compounds—such as diallyl disulfide and diallyl trisulfide—that have demonstrated an-ti-inflammatory, antimicrobial, and cardioprotective properties (Amagase et al., 2001). These sulfur compounds can modulate the inflammatory process by inhibiting the production and re-lease of pro-inflammatory cytokines, including TNF-α and IL-1β, thereby tempering the immune system's tendency to remain in a perpetually elevated state of alert (Bayan et al., 2014).

Several lines of evidence point to garlic's ability to reduce ox-idative stress, an underlying driver of long-standing inflamma-tion. By scavenging free radicals and supporting antioxidant enzyme systems, garlic lowers the likelihood that these unsta-ble molecules will damage cells and provoke an inflammatory reaction (Banerjee et al., 2003). Animal models of conditions like atherosclerosis often show that adding garlic to the diet can reduce plaque development, in part by mitigating the in-flammatory events that contribute to artery damage (Sobenin et al., 2010). Similarly, human trials have observed that garlic supplementation can modestly lower markers like C-reactive protein (CRP), which is often elevated in chronic inflammation (Dhawan and Jain, 2005).

Interestingly, garlic can also affect the behaviour of white blood cells, which are key players in immune and inflamma-tory processes. Certain studies suggest that garlic extracts or constituents can reduce leukocyte adhesion and migration to sites of inflammation (El-Batayneh et al., 2020). While these immune cells are necessary for acute inflammatory responses, excessive or uncontrolled movement into tissues can worsen damage. By encouraging a more balanced, measured immune response, garlic helps the body resolve inflammation more ef-fectively once a threat has passed.

Another area of interest is the link between garlic and met-abolic health. Chronic inflammation is often intertwined with conditions such as insulin resistance, obesity, and metabolic syndrome. Garlic may help by improving insulin sensitivity and influencing lipid metabolism, which indirectly dampens inflammatory processes (Asdaq et al., 2022). Indeed, high levels of circulating free fatty acids and dysfunctional lipids can incite inflammatory pathways, so any dietary measure that nudges lipids and glucose toward normal ranges will typically have a downstream effect on inflammation.

Incorporating garlic into daily meals is a simple way to access these benefits. Fresh garlic, particularly when chopped or crushed and allowed to sit briefly before cooking, offers a higher concentration of allicin. Overcooking can degrade some of the beneficial sulfur compounds, so short cooking times or raw uses (such as in pestos or dressings) can preserve potency. Some individuals who find raw garlic too overpowering might opt for aged garlic extracts or odour-controlled supplements, which can still harbour many of the anti-inflammatory compounds without the pungent smell. Even so, moderation and personal tolerance should guide intake. Garlic can sometimes irritate the digestive tract or interact with medications that affect blood thinning, so it's wise to pay attention to one's body and consult a healthcare practitioner for more personalised guidance.

Ginger

Ginger (*Zingiber officinale*) is another spice with an unmistakable flavour: a hint of peppery heat softened by a sweet, woody undertone. It appears as a staple ingredient in countless dishes and beverages, from stir-fries to herbal teas. Traditionally, ginger has been relied upon to soothe an upset stomach, enhance circulation, and bolster overall vitality (Grzanna et al., 2005). It is only in the last few decades, however, that researchers have begun unraveling the complexity of ginger's biochemical profile and its notable anti-inflammatory capabilities.

The phytochemicals responsible for ginger's characteristic taste and effects are collectively known as gingerols and shogaols, with **[6]-gingerol** frequently singled out for its relevance to inflammation (Ali et al., 2008). Much like the bioactive constituents of turmeric and garlic, these compounds target multiple pathways. They can suppress the activation of NF-κB, thus curbing the production of pro-inflammatory cytokines (TNF-α, IL-6) and enzymes (COX-2) that perpetuate inflammation (Grzanna et al., 2005). In this way, ginger appears to work in parallel to turmeric, albeit with different molecular actors.

Another mechanism, increasingly recognised, involves ginger's antioxidant action. By quenching reactive oxygen species, ginger reduces oxidative stress that typically sets the stage for prolonged inflammatory responses (Rahmani et al., 2014). Cells under oxidative stress often release distress signals that beckon immune cells and trigger further inflammation. Ginger's capacity to calm that initial spark can keep the process from escalating in the first place.

Human clinical trials have provided some of the more compelling evidence for ginger's role in reducing inflammation-related symptoms. For instance, multiple studies on osteoarthritis have shown that ginger supplementation can lessen pain and swelling in the joints (Altman and Marcussen, 2001). These effects may appear subtle compared to pharmaceutical anti-inflammatory drugs, but ginger is rarely associated with significant adverse effects or gastric distress, which makes it an appealing long-term option for certain populations. In addition, those dealing with exercise-induced muscle soreness have found that ginger can reduce both the intensity and duration of post-exercise inflammation (Black and O'Connor, 2010). It seems that whether inflammation stems from metabolic dysfunction, autoimmune challenges, or simple mechanical stress, ginger can help restore equilibrium.

Much like turmeric, ginger also intersects with metabolic health. Chronic inflammation can arise when there is insulin resistance, high blood lipids, or excessive adipose tissue. Research indicates that ginger might help increase insulin sensitivity and stabilise blood glucose levels (Mahluji et al., 2013).

While more extensive studies are required, the preliminary evidence suggests that ginger's impact on inflammatory mediators extends to many facets of metabolic regulation. Essentially, ginger's anti-inflammatory benefits can ripple outward, influencing broader aspects of health in a supportive, integrative manner.

From a culinary standpoint, ginger's versatility makes it easy to incorporate into diverse dishes. Fresh ginger root can be grated or sliced into soups, stir-fries, or even smoothies, adding a zesty kick while imparting protective phytochemicals. Dried and powdered ginger is convenient for baked goods, spice blends, or even sprinkled into herbal teas. Many cultures have also embraced pickled or candied ginger. Although the candying process involves sugar, it still retains traces of ginger's active compounds. For maximum potency, however, using fresh or minimally processed ginger is often recommended, as prolonged heat or excessive processing can degrade the delicate gingerols.

Cinnamon

Cinnamon is one of the most beloved and widely used spices worldwide. Its characteristic aroma and warm flavour come primarily from an essential compound called cinnamaldehyde (Shan et al., 2005). While it is often associated with desserts and sweet treats, its health benefits are increasingly recognised in scientific literature, particularly for its anti-inflammatory and antioxidant potential (Sadeghi et al., 2014).

One of the key ways cinnamon may influence inflammatory pathways is through the inhibition of specific molecules known as pro-inflammatory cytokines. These cytokines—like interleukin-6 (IL-6) and tumour necrosis factor-alpha (TNF-α)—are heavily involved in amplifying inflammation. Research indicates that extracts of cinnamon may help reduce the production of these pro-inflammatory cytokines, thereby modulating the body's immune response (Cao et al., 2018). In addition, cinnamaldehyde has been shown to inhibit the nuclear factor kappa B (NF-κB) signalling pathway (Imparl-Radosevich et al., 1998). NF-κB is a major regulator of inflammation and is implicated in many chronic inflammatory conditions. By keeping NF-κB in check, cinnamon may help to prevent the runaway train of inflammation that leads to tissue damage over time.

Another mechanism behind cinnamon's anti-inflammatory action is its antioxidant capacity. Many chronic inflammatory conditions are associated with an excess of free radicals—unstable molecules that damage cells and tissues (Cao et al., 2018). Cinnamon contains polyphenolic compounds that can help neutralise these free radicals, limiting the oxidative stress that often triggers or worsens inflammation (Shan et al., 2005).

Cinnamon's benefits aren't limited to laboratory findings. Human clinical trials have begun to explore its role in managing metabolic markers of inflammation. For instance, individuals with type 2 diabetes or metabolic syndrome frequently exhibit elevated inflammatory markers, such as C-reactive protein (CRP). One study found that supplementation with cinnamon led to reductions in CRP, suggesting a potential role in mitigating low-grade chronic inflammation (Zare et al., 2019). While more large-scale clinical trials are needed for a definitive conclusion, the evidence so far is promising enough to consider cinnamon a valuable spice in an anti-inflammatory diet.

Clove

Cloves are the dried flower buds of the *Syzygium aromaticum* tree and hold a prominent place in traditional medicine and culinary traditions. Their anti-inflammatory properties are primarily linked to a compound called eugenol (Cortés-Rojas et al., 2014). Eugenol imparts that characteristic pungent, warm flavour that makes cloves so recognisable.

At the cellular level, eugenol appears to interact with several inflammatory mediators. It can reduce the synthesis of prostaglandins, which are hormone-like substances that mediate inflammatory and pain signals (Chaieb et al., 2007). This mechanism is akin to certain non-steroidal anti-inflammatory drugs (NSAIDs), though on a much gentler scale. Clove's natural capacity to modulate prostaglandins may explain why clove oil is traditionally used for toothache or joint pain, both of which involve local inflammation.

Moreover, cloves boast a high antioxidant activity, often ranking near the top in tests measuring the total antioxidant content of various spices (Shan et al., 2005). These antioxidants help to scavenge free radicals, reducing the oxidative stress that feeds into chronic inflammatory pathways (Lee & Balick, 2005). Because chronic inflammation often involves a vicious cycle of oxidative damage and immune activation, using cloves in cooking or as part of herbal remedies can contribute to breaking that loop.

Beyond eugenol, cloves contain flavonoids and other bioactive compounds that may complement eugenol's anti-inflammatory effects. Some studies have reported reductions in both TNF-α and IL-6 in animal models given clove extracts (Rasool & Varalakshmi, 2006). While human trials are still somewhat limited, preliminary data indicate that clove could serve as a supportive element for overall inflammatory balance, particularly when integrated into a broader anti-inflammatory diet.

Black Pepper

Black pepper is a staple in almost every kitchen, but its significance extends beyond taste. The compound piperine, responsible for black pepper's pungent bite, has been extensively investigated for its anti-inflammatory and anti-oxidant activities (Meghwal & Goswami, 2012). Piperine's major mechanism of action involves the modulation of cytokine production and the inhibition of NF-κB (Srinivasan, 2007), similar to what we see with cinnamaldehyde in cinnamon.

One particularly interesting aspect of black pepper is its ability to enhance bioavailability of other compounds. For instance, black pepper is often combined with turmeric in formulations because piperine has been shown to increase the absorption of curcumin (the active component in turmeric) by up to 2,000% (Shoba et al., 1998). This synergy not only intensifies black pepper's anti-inflammatory credentials but also points to its role as a booster for other anti-inflammatory agents.

In terms of practical application, black pepper's effect on inflammation is subtle but consistent. Animal studies have demonstrated that piperine can reduce oedema (swelling due to inflammation) and lower levels of inflammatory markers in serum (Srinivasan, 2007). Some preliminary clinical data suggest that supplementation with piperine-containing extracts can alleviate mild inflammation and support healthy immune function (Meghwal & Goswami, 2012).

Cayenne Pepper

Cayenne pepper, part of the broader family of chilli peppers, owes its heat to capsaicin. Capsaicin is famous for creating a burning sensation on the tongue, but it is also valued for its anti-inflammatory properties (Joo & Jung, 2014). This compound primarily works by interacting with TRPV1 receptors, which are sensory neurons responsible for pain and heat sensation. While capsaicin is known as a topical analgesic (it's often found in creams for muscle and joint pain), its anti-inflammatory effects are not limited to topical use.

From a biochemical standpoint, capsaicin can reduce the expression of pro-inflammatory cytokines, including IL-6 and TNF-α (Lee et al., 2013). By dampening these cytokines, cayenne pepper contributes to the regulation of inflammatory processes in a similar manner to other chilli peppers. Furthermore, chilli peppers, including cayenne, possess antioxidants that protect cells from oxidative stress (Bae et al., 2014).

Additionally, some evidence suggests that capsaicin can help support metabolic health by improving insulin sensitivity and reducing the risk of obesity-related inflammation (Whiting et al., 2012). Chronic inflammation is often intertwined with metabolic dysfunction, making cayenne pepper potentially beneficial on multiple fronts. However, it's important to remember that cayenne pepper's pungency can be a limiting factor for some individuals. Gradual introduction into the diet is often recommended.

Paprika

Paprika is a ground spice derived from dried red peppers (often variants of *Capsicum annuum*). Its vibrant red colour points to a rich content of carotenoids, notably capsanthin and capsorubin, which contribute to its antioxidant and possibly anti-inflammatory effects (Topuz & Ozdemir, 2007).

Although paprika tends to be milder than cayenne pepper, it still contains a level of capsaicinoids, the family of compounds that includes capsaicin. Studies show that even moderate levels of capsaicinoids can help to suppress inflammatory signalling by reducing the production of TNF-α and IL-1β (Ma et al., 2015). Paprika's carotenoids also play a role in quenching free radicals, reducing the oxidative stress that can exacerbate chronic inflammation (Kim et al., 2011).

Paprika's flavour profile ranges from sweet to very spicy, depending on the type of peppers used. Both sweet and hot varieties can contribute to managing inflammation, but the hotter versions contain more capsaicinoids. The availability of paprika in various heat levels makes it an accessible option for those who are sensitive to spiciness yet still wish to reap some anti-inflammatory benefits.

Other Notable Anti-Inflammatory Spices

Cardamom

Cardamom, known for its sweet and spicy aroma, contains terpenes and other volatile oils that demonstrate anti-inflammatory and antioxidant activities (Jafari et al., 2017). Some studies show that cardamom supplementation can reduce levels of C-reactive protein and lipid peroxidation in patients with metabolic syndrome, pointing to an overall improvement in inflammatory status (Sundaresan et al., 2013).

Cumin

Cumin seeds are a staple in various global cuisines. The key active compounds include cuminaldehyde and terpenoids, which have been linked to reduced production of inflammatory mediators (Gharby et al., 2014). Additionally, cumin's antioxidant capacity can help safeguard cells from oxidative stress, contributing to a balanced inflammatory response (Sharma et al., 2020).

Coriander

Coriander seeds have a long history in both culinary and medicinal contexts. These seeds are rich in linalool and linoleic acid, which exhibit anti-inflammatory properties by down regulating certain cytokines (Warrier et al., 2021). Animal studies have shown that coriander seed extract can mitigate inflammation and oxidative damage in various disease models, suggesting a supportive role in maintaining healthy inflammatory pathways.

Fennel Seeds

Fennel seeds stand out for their anethole content—a compound linked to anti-inflammatory and antispasmodic effects

(Faudale et al., 2008). These seeds not only offer digestive comfort but also help modulate the levels of pro-inflammatory enzymes like cyclooxygenase-2 (COX-2). By inhibiting these enzymes, fennel seeds can reduce the synthesis of pro-inflammatory prostaglandins, thereby easing inflammation.

Fenugreek

Fenugreek seeds are another treasure trove of phytochemicals, including trigonelline and diosgenin, both of which are recognised for their anti-inflammatory and metabolic benefits (Basch et al., 2003). Clinical trials have reported improvements in glycemic control and reductions in inflammatory markers when fenugreek is included in the diet (Neelakantan et al., 2014). Since chronic inflammation and insulin resistance often go hand in hand, fenugreek can be a valuable ally in supporting both metabolic and inflammatory health.

Mustard Seeds

Mustard seeds, particularly the brown and black varieties, are rich in glucosinolates which convert into isothiocyanates upon crushing or grinding (Fahey et al., 2001). Isothiocyanates are known to have anti-inflammatory and anticancerproperties by modulating inflammatory pathways and detoxification enzymes (Traka & Mithen, 2009). Their pungent flavor is also a signal of their biologically active constituents that can help protect cells from damage and reduce inflammation.

Star Anise

Star anise is renowned for its anethole content, much like fennel seeds, giving it a sweet, licorice-like flavour. This compound is credited with anti-inflammatory properties through the inhibition of cytokines and enzymes that promote inflammation (Peter & Gandhi, 2017). Additionally, star anise contains shikimic acid, which has been studied for its potential antiviral and immunomodulatory effects (Yang et al., 2015). Together, these compounds make star anise a valuable spice for managing inflammation and supporting overall immune health.

Less Common but Potent Anti-Inflammatory Spices

Saffron

Often regarded as the world's most expensive spice, saffron is derived from the stigmas of the *Crocus sativus* flower. Its high price tag is due to the labor-intensive harvesting process. Key bioactive components in saffron include crocin and safranal, both of which have demonstrated anti-inflammatory and antioxidant properties (Poma et al., 2012). These compounds may help reduce levels of prostaglandins and cytokines, thereby limiting the inflammatory cascade. Human trials suggest saffron may alleviate symptoms in conditions like mild depression and metabolic syndrome, both of which can be exacerbated by chronic inflammation (Kashani et al., 2018).

Nutmeg

Nutmeg comes from the seed of the *Myristica fragrans* tree and is known for its warm, sweet aroma. The main active components—myristicin and macelignan—contribute to its anti-inflammatory and antioxidant effects (Piaru et al., 2012). Studies indicate that nutmeg extracts can inhibit nitric oxide and prostaglandin production, which are crucial mediators in inflammatory processes (Olajide et al., 2009). Its strong flavor profile means a small amount goes a long way, making it easy to incorporate into both sweet and savory dishes.

Bay Leaves

Bay leaves, harvested from the bay laurel tree (*Laurus nobilis*), contain compounds such as eucalyptol, linalool, and other volatile oils that exhibit anti-inflammatory actions by reducing cytokine levels (Elbetieha et al., 2014). In addition, bay leaves can help regulate lipid metabolism, which is relevant since unhealthy lipid profiles can be closely intertwined with inflammation. Some traditional remedies also suggest using bay leaf tea for digestive complaints—a domain where inflammation often plays a role.

Sumac

Sumac is a tangy, deep-red spice widely used in Middle Eastern cuisine. It contains high levels of polyphenols, including gallic acid and quercetin, that contribute to its potent antioxidant capacity (Güllüce et al., 2004). By mitigating oxidative stress, sumac can indirectly help control inflammatory pathways, making it a noteworthy spice for people aiming to optimise their diet for lower inflammation. Preliminary studies in animal models also suggest sumac may help lower inflammatory mediators and improve blood lipid profiles (Gündoğdu, 2012).

Allspice

Allspice, derived from the dried berries of *Pimenta dioica*, combines the flavours of cinnamon, nutmeg, and cloves all in one. The primary active compounds, like eugenol (as found in cloves) and quercetin, offer anti-inflammatory and antioxidant benefits (Bahamondes et al., 2016). These compounds can block the release of pro-inflammatory cytokines and may also reduce oxidative damage to tissues. Although allspice is more commonly associated with baking or Christmas-themed dishes in some cultures, it is used year-round in Caribbean and Latin American cuisines for meats, stews, and sauces. These broader applications make it another diverse and tasty way to support a balanced inflammatory response.

Synergistic Effects and Practical Considerations

In most cuisines worldwide, spices are rarely used in isolation. Instead, they are combined in endless variations—think of garam masala, ras el hanout, five-spice powder, or even a simple spice rub for grilling. This blending often delivers synergistic benefits, where the combined anti-inflammatory effects of multiple spices can exceed the sum of their parts (Aggarwal & Shishodia, 2006). For example, the synergy between black pepper and other spices like turmeric has already been noted, but similar principles apply to many of the spices discussed here.

It's also important to remember practical considerations:

1. **Dosage and Frequency**: While these spices can offer health benefits, they need to be consumed consistently in meaningful amounts to exert a noticeable physiological effect. Regularly incorporating them into your diet—sprinkling cinnamon on oatmeal, adding paprika to roasted vegetables, or making spice blends for marinades—ensures you keep the inflammatory fires in check.

2. **Quality and Storage**: Spices lose potency over time, especially if they are ground. The active compounds degrade with prolonged exposure to air, light, and heat. It is wise to buy whole spices where possible (like whole nutmegs or peppercorns), then grind them fresh to preserve their bioactive components. Proper storage in airtight containers away from direct sunlight can also help maintain potency.

3. **Synergies with Whole Foods**: While spices are powerful, they are most effective when part of a broader, nutrient-dense diet rich in fruits, vegetables, whole grains, and healthy fats. The vitamins, minerals, and phytochemicals found in whole foods create a supportive environment for these anti-inflammatory spices to do their work.

4. **Potential Interactions**: Some spices—particularly those with strong bioactive compounds—can interact with med-

ications or existing health conditions. For instance, high doses of cinnamon might affect blood sugar regulation, and black pepper may increase the absorption of certain drugs, thus altering their effective dose (Shoba et al., 1998). It's always best to consult a healthcare professional if you have concerns.

The Plan & Recipes

Now that you have all of the science and the fundamentals of the plan nailed, its time to put it all into practice. I know that there may well be a lot to take in and a lot of complex information to process but, as you will see, putting into practice is actually extremely easy and also a delicious and enjoyable way to live.

Your 6 Week Eating Plan

Day	Breakfast	Lunch	Dinner	Snack
Week 1, Day 1	Spicy Scrambled Tofu with Spinach, Turmeric, and Chilli	Courgette Fritters with Tzatziki	Sweet Potato & Chickpea Coconut Curry	Olive Tapenade with Crudités
Week 1, Day 2	Baked Sweet Potato with Walnuts, Cinnamon, and Greek Yogurt	Smoked Mackerel & Watercress Soup	Baked Salmon with Walnut & Herb Crust	Beetroot & Goat's Cheese Bites
Week 1, Day 3	Sardine & Avocado Wrap with Cucumber and Lemon	Mushroom & Spinach Omelette	Baked Trout with Caper & Dill Butter	Olive Tapenade with Crudités
Week 1, Day 4	Omega Porridge with Walnuts, Cinnamon & Berries	Stuffed Peppers with Quinoa & Herbs	Cod with Puy Lentils & Mustard Dressing	Stuffed Dates with Almond Butter

Week 1, Day 5	Coconut & Cinnamon Chia Porridge with Berries	Spiced Lentil & Beetroot Salad	Baked Salmon with Walnut & Herb Crust	Stuffed Dates with Almond Butter
Week 1, Day 6	Coconut & Cinnamon Chia Porridge with Berries	Roasted Garlic & Celeriac Soup	Grilled Lamb Chops with Mint & Garlic	Homemade Flaxseed Granola Clusters
Week 1, Day 7	Turmeric & Herb Poached Eggs with Avocado and Spinach Salad	Leek, Fennel & Salmon Chowder	Stuffed Butternut Squash with Quinoa & Pumpkin Seeds	Flax & Chia Seed Crackers
Week 2, Day 1	Coconut & Cinnamon Chia Porridge with Berries	Cucumber & Avocado Chilled Soup	Baked Salmon with Walnut & Herb Crust	Olive Tapenade with Crudités
Week 2, Day 2	Smoked Salmon & Avocado Omelette with Dill and Lemon	Curried Cauliflower & Lentil Salad	Braised Lamb Shoulder with Garlic & Rosemary	Curried Roasted Chickpeas
Week 2, Day 3	Flaxseed & Berry Smoothie with Ginger	Leek, Fennel & Salmon Chowder	Grilled Lamb Chops with Mint & Garlic	Chia & Almond Butter Energy Balls
Week 2, Day 4	Smoked Salmon & Avocado Omelette with Dill and Lemon	Smoked Mackerel & Watercress Soup	Cod & Spinach Coconut Curry	Olive Tapenade with Crudités
Week 2, Day 5	Coconut & Cinnamon Chia Porridge with Berries	Pumpkin & Red Lentil Soup	Turmeric-Spiced Chicken & Cauliflower Rice	Turmeric-Spiced Nuts
Week 2, Day 6	Coconut & Cinnamon Chia Porridge with Berries	Spiced Lentil & Beetroot Salad	Spicy Turkey & Spinach Meatballs	Smoked Salmon & Cucumber Bites
Week 2, Day 7	Omega Porridge with Walnuts, Cinnamon & Berries	Spinach & Walnut Pesto Courgetti	Cod with Puy Lentils & Mustard Dressing	Homemade Flaxseed Granola Clusters

Week 3, Day 1	Smoked Salmon & Avocado Omelette with Dill and Lemon	Butternut Squash & Sage Soup	Baked Salmon with Walnut & Herb Crust	Curried Roasted Chickpeas
Week 3, Day 2	Flaxseed & Berry Smoothie with Ginger	Mushroom & Spinach Omelette	Slow-Cooked Beef & Mushroom Stew	Homemade Flaxseed Granola Clusters
Week 3, Day 3	Turmeric & Herb Poached Eggs with Avocado and Spinach Salad	Beetroot & Ginger Soup	Lentil & Aubergine Moussaka	Turmeric-Spiced Roasted Almonds
Week 3, Day 4	Omega Porridge with Walnuts, Cinnamon & Berries	Stuffed Peppers with Quinoa & Herbs	Spicy Turkey & Spinach Meatballs	Walnut & Dark Chocolate Bites
Week 3, Day 5	Omega Porridge with Walnuts, Cinnamon & Berries	Spicy Roasted Tomato & Basil Soup	Cod & Spinach Coconut Curry	Stuffed Dates with Almond Butter
Week 3, Day 6	Omega Porridge with Walnuts, Cinnamon & Berries	Butternut Squash & Sage Soup	Stuffed Butternut Squash with Quinoa & Pumpkin Seeds	Beetroot & Goat's Cheese Bites
Week 3, Day 7	Sardine & Avocado Wrap with Cucumber and Lemon	Broccoli, Kale & Almond Soup	Turmeric-Spiced Chicken & Cauliflower Rice	Tahini & Cinnamon Energy Bars
Week 4, Day 1	Omega Porridge with Walnuts, Cinnamon & Berries	Pea & Mint Soup with Omega-3 Drizzle	Braised Lamb Shoulder with Garlic & Rosemary	Tahini & Cinnamon Energy Bars
Week 4, Day 2	Omega Porridge with Walnuts, Cinnamon & Berries	Roasted Garlic & Celeriac Soup	Cod & Spinach Coconut Curry	Walnut & Dark Chocolate Bites

Week 4, Day 3	Omega Porridge with Walnuts, Cinnamon & Berries	Chickpea & Red Pepper Hummus Bowl	Roast Chicken with Lemon & Thyme	Stuffed Dates with Almond Butter
Week 4, Day 4	Sardine & Avocado Wrap with Cucumber and Lemon	Grilled Aubergine with Walnut Salsa	Cod & Spinach Coconut Curry	Smoked Salmon & Cucumber Bites
Week 4, Day 5	Turmeric & Herb Poached Eggs with Avocado and Spinach Salad	Smoked Mackerel & Watercress Soup	Turmeric-Spiced Chicken & Cauliflower Rice	Stuffed Dates with Almond Butter
Week 4, Day 6	Chia & Flaxseed Pudding with Walnuts and Blueberry Compote	Salmon & Avocado Wraps	Spicy Turkey & Spinach Meatballs	Smoked Salmon & Cucumber Bites
Week 4, Day 7	Baked Sweet Potato with Walnuts, Cinnamon, and Greek Yogurt	Spicy Roasted Tomato & Basil Soup	Slow-Cooked Beef & Mushroom Stew	Stuffed Dates with Almond Butter
Week 5, Day 1	Mackerel & Avocado Omelette with Lemon and Turmeric	Turmeric-Spiced Cauliflower Soup	Baked Salmon with Walnut & Herb Crust	Tahini & Cinnamon Energy Bars
Week 5, Day 2	Baked Sweet Potato with Walnuts, Cinnamon, and Greek Yogurt	Butternut Squash & Sage Soup	Spicy Turkey & Spinach Meatballs	Tahini & Cinnamon Energy Bars
Week 5, Day 3	Baked Sweet Potato with Walnuts, Cinnamon, and Greek Yogurt	Beetroot & Ginger Soup	Lentil & Aubergine Moussaka	Stuffed Dates with Almond Butter
Week 5, Day 4	Baked Sweet Potato with Walnuts, Cinnamon, and Greek Yogurt	Leek, Fennel & Salmon Chowder	Grilled Lamb Chops with Mint & Garlic	Avocado & Cacao Mousse

Week 5, Day 5	Omega Porridge with Walnuts, Cinnamon & Berries	Butternut Squash & Sage Soup	Grilled Lamb Chops with Mint & Garlic	Homemade Flaxseed Granola Clusters
Week 5, Day 6	Mackerel & Avocado Omelette with Lemon and Turmeric	Asparagus & Lemon Soup	Beef & Cabbage Stir-Fry	Turmeric-Spiced Roasted Almonds
Week 5, Day 7	Spicy Scrambled Tofu with Spinach, Turmeric, and Chilli	Chickpea & Red Pepper Hummus Bowl	Beef & Cabbage Stir-Fry	Olive Tapenade with Crudités
Week 6, Day 1	Sardine & Avocado Wrap with Cucumber and Lemon	Spicy Roasted Tomato & Basil Soup	Rosemary & Garlic Roasted Duck Breast	Stuffed Dates with Almond Butter
Week 6, Day 2	Turmeric & Herb Poached Eggs with Avocado and Spinach Salad	Curried Cauliflower & Lentil Salad	Grilled Lamb Chops with Mint & Garlic	Curried Roasted Chickpeas
Week 6, Day 3	Omega Porridge with Walnuts, Cinnamon & Berries	Roasted Broccoli & Almond Salad	Slow-Cooked Beef & Mushroom Stew	Flax & Chia Seed Crackers
Week 6, Day 4	Turmeric & Herb Poached Eggs with Avocado and Spinach Salad	Curried Parsnip & Coconut Soup	Rosemary & Garlic Roasted Duck Breast	Stuffed Dates with Almond Butter
Week 6, Day 5	Flaxseed & Berry Smoothie with Ginger	Pea & Mint Soup with Omega-3 Drizzle	Sweet Potato & Chickpea Coconut Curry	Curried Roasted Chickpeas
Week 6, Day 6	Mackerel & Avocado Omelette with Lemon and Turmeric	Spiced Lentil & Beetroot Salad	Baked Trout with Caper & Dill Butter	Flax & Chia Seed Crackers
Week 6, Day 7	Mackerel & Avocado Omelette with Lemon and Turmeric	Turmeric-Spiced Cauliflower Soup	Rosemary & Garlic Roasted Duck Breast	Smoked Salmon & Cucumber Bites

How you start your day matters! It really matters. It is time to drop the sugary, processed cereal and toast. There is a whole new world of breakfast options. This first section will definitely have you covered.

Chia & Flaxseed Pudding with Walnuts and Blueberry Compote

Ok, so chia puddings may be a little bit 'Instagram', but there is a good reason why they have become so popular. They are quick, easy and absolutely delicious.

Ingredients

» 2 tbsp chia seeds
» 1 tbsp ground flaxseeds
» 150ml unsweetened almond milk
» 1 tbsp maple syrup (optional)
» 30g walnuts, chopped
» 100g fresh blueberries
» 1 tsp lemon zest
» 1 tsp ground cinnamon

Method

» Combine the chia seeds, flaxseeds, almond milk, and maple syrup in a bowl.
» Stir well and let it set in the fridge overnight.
» For the compote, cook the blueberries and lemon zest in a pan on low heat for 5 minutes, then stir in cinnamon.
» Top the pudding with the blueberry compote and chopped walnuts in the morning.

Turmeric & Herb Poached Eggs with Avocado and Spinach Salad

Salad for breakfast! Yes. It's a thing. It may seem a little odd at first, but that is just because of how we have been conditioned. Remember, one of the absolute keys to this plan is to maximise our intake of non starchy, brightly coloured veg, packed with all of those anti-inflammatory chemicals. This is how we do it!

Ingredients

» 2 large eggs
» 1 tsp turmeric
» 30g spinach
» 1/2 avocado, sliced

» 1 tbsp olive oil
» 1/2 tsp ground black pepper
» Fresh herbs

Preparation

» Poach the eggs in simmering water with a pinch of turmeric for 3-4 minutes.
» While the eggs are poaching, sauté the spinach in olive oil until wilted, then toss with fresh herbs.
» Arrange the poached eggs on a plate with avocado slices, drizzle with olive oil, and serve alongside the spinach salad.

Omega Porridge with Walnuts, Cinnamon & Berries

Porridge, but upgraded. This dish relies o plant sources of omega 3 which, may not be as powerful as EPA & DHA, but still help to reduce inflammation.

Ingredients

» 40g rolled oats
» 1 tbsp ground flaxseeds
» 150ml unsweetened almond milk
» 30g walnuts, chopped

» 100g mixed berries (blueberries, raspberries, strawberries)
» 1/2 tsp cinnamon
» 1 tbsp chia seeds
» Stevia or honey to taste

Method

» Cook the oats with almond milk until creamy, then stir in ground flaxseeds and chia seeds.
» Top with walnuts, fresh berries, a dash of cinnamon, and sweetener to taste.

Smoked Salmon & Avocado Omelette with Dill and Lemon

Omelettes are an absolute staple of the anti-inflammatory lifestyle as they are a low glycemic dish, and a great vehicle to pack out with potent anti-inflammatory ingredients.

Ingredients

» 2 large eggs
» 50g smoked salmon
» 1/2 avocado, sliced
» 1 tbsp olive oil
» 1 tsp fresh dill
» Squeeze of lemon

Method

» Whisk the eggs and pour into a hot pan with olive oil.
» Once the eggs begin to set, add the smoked salmon, avocado slices, and dill to one side.
» Fold the omelette over and cook for another 1-2 minutes. Serve with a squeeze of lemon juice on top.

Baked Sweet Potato with Walnuts, Cinnamon, and Greek Yogurt

I haven't lost my mind. I promise you! I first experienced incorporating sweet potatoes into sweeter dishes when I lived in Japan. It works. It really works. try it.

Ingredients

» 1 medium sweet potato
» 30g walnuts, chopped
» 1 tsp cinnamon

» 150g Greek yogurt (full-fat or low-fat)
» 1 tsp honey (optional)

Method

» Bake the sweet potato at 180°C for 40-45 minutes or until soft.
» Once baked, slice it open and top with chopped walnuts, cinnamon, and a dollop of Greek yogurt.
» Drizzle with honey for added sweetness.

Coconut & Cinnamon Chia Porridge with Berries

Another beautifully simple morning staple.

Ingredients

» 2 tbsp chia seeds
» 150ml coconut milk (unsweetened)
» 1/4 tsp ground cinnamon
» 100g mixed berries
» 1 tbsp ground flaxseeds
» 1 tbsp desiccated coconut

Method

» Mix the chia seeds, coconut milk, ground cinnamon, and flax-seeds in a bowl.
» Let it sit in the fridge overnight.
» In the morning, top the chia pudding with mixed berries and desiccated coconut for an extra burst of anti-inflammatory goodness.

Sardine & Avocado Wrap with Cucumber and Lemon

This is a great on the go recipe that can be made in minutes and then grabbed as you run out of the door.

Ingredients

» 1 can (100g) sardines in olive oil
» 1/2 avocado, sliced
» 1 small cucumber, thinly sliced
» 1 whole wheat or rye wrap
» Juice of 1/2 lemon
» Fresh parsley, chopped

Method

» Warm the wrap slightly, then layer the sardines, avocado, cucumber slices, and parsley.
» Drizzle with lemon juice, wrap it up, and enjoy a fibre-packed, omega-3-rich breakfast.

Spicy Scrambled Tofu with Spinach, Turmeric, and Chilli

Scrambled tofu is a thing. Who'd have thought? It works very well if you want a high protein breakfast

Ingredients

» 150g firm tofu, crumbled
» 30g spinach
» 1/2 tsp turmeric
» 1/4 tsp ground chilli
» 1 tbsp olive oil
» 1/2 tbsp tamari sauce (or soy sauce)
» Fresh coriander to garnish

Method

» Heat olive oil in a pan, add the crumbled tofu and turmeric, and stir-fry for 2-3 minutes. Add spinach and cook until wilted. Stir in tamari sauce and ground chilli for extra flavour. Garnish with fresh coriander and serve.

Flaxseed & Berry Smoothie with Ginger

Im not often a fan of smoothies unless they are done right. Generally they are sugar packed and send blood glucose through the roof. This has a lot more fibre and protein, so will buffer the release of the natural sugars.

Ingredients

» 1 tbsp ground flaxseeds
» 50g silken tofu
» 150g frozen mixed berries (blueberries, raspberries, strawberries)
» 1/2 banana (for sweetness)
» 1/2 tsp ground ginger
» 200ml unsweetened almond milk
» 1 tbsp almond butter

Method

» Blend all ingredients together until smooth.
» Serve chilled.

Mackerel & Avocado Omelette with Lemon and Turmeric

A beautiful flavoursome omelette that will keep you full and is packed with all the right stuff!

Ingredients

» 2 large eggs
» 1 can (100g) mackerel in olive oil
» 1/2 avocado, sliced
» 1 tsp olive oil
» 1/2 tsp turmeric
» Fresh parsley or dill, chopped
» Juice of 1/2 lemon
» Ground black pepper

Method

» Heat the olive oil in a non-stick pan over medium heat.
» While the pan is heating, crack the eggs into a bowl, whisk them together, and season with a pinch of black pepper and the turmeric.
» Pour the egg mixture into the pan and let it set for about 1-2 minutes.
» Once the edges begin to firm up, add the mackerel (drained and flaked), sliced avocado, and fresh herbs to one half of the omelette.
» Gently fold the omelette over the filling and cook for another 2-3 minutes until the eggs are fully set.
» Serve with a squeeze of lemon juice on top for an extra burst of flavour.

There is just something so satisfying about a delicious, comforting soup. A perfect lunchtime companion and an easy thing to make ahead to last you a few days. Also, starters. If you love having a three course meal, are entertaining friends, or just want lighter meals, then you are covered.

Turmeric-Spiced Cauliflower Soup

This is an absolutely stunning dish and one that I used to make often back in around 2003 whilst I was at University and was working in the kitchen of a local student pub. A creamy, warming soup packed with anti-inflammatory turmeric and gut-friendly cauliflower. Feeding the microbiome never tasted so good.

Ingredients

» 1 medium cauliflower, chopped into florets
» 1 onion, finely chopped
» 2 cloves garlic, minced
» 1-inch piece ginger, grated
» 1 tsp turmeric
» ½ tsp ground cumin
» ½ tsp ground coriander
» 800ml vegetable stock
» 200ml coconut milk
» 1 tbsp olive oil
» Sea salt & black pepper, to taste
» Fresh coriander, to garnish

Method

» Heat the olive oil in a large saucepan over medium heat. Add the onion and sauté for 5 minutes until softened.
» Add the garlic and ginger, cooking for another minute until fragrant.
» Stir in the turmeric, cumin, and coriander. Cook for 30 seconds.
» Add the cauliflower and stock. Bring to a boil, then simmer for 15 minutes until the cauliflower is tender.

- » Stir in the coconut milk, then blend the soup until smooth using a hand blender.
- » Season with salt and pepper. Serve garnished with fresh coriander.

Smoked Mackerel & Watercress Soup

Ok, I know this sounds a little bit....weird...but stick with me on this. A rich, long chain omega-3-packed soup with a peppery kick from watercress.

Ingredients

» 2 fillets smoked mackerel, skin removed, flaked
» 1 large onion, finely chopped
» 1 leek, finely sliced
» 2 cloves garlic, minced
» 1 medium potato, peeled and diced
» 700ml fish or vegetable stock
» 150g watercress
» 200ml unsweetened almond milk
» 1 tbsp olive oil
» Sea salt & black pepper, to taste
» Lemon wedges, to serve

Method

» Heat the olive oil in a large saucepan and sauté the onion and leek for 5 minutes until soft.
» Add the garlic and potato, then pour in the stock. Simmer for 15 minutes until the potato is tender.
» Stir in the watercress and almond milk. Cook for 2 minutes.
» Blend the soup until smooth, then stir in the smoked mackerel.
» Season to taste and serve with lemon wedges.

Roasted Garlic & Celeriac Soup

This is an incredible food source for our gut microbiome. The inulin in the garlic and the multitude of fibres in the celeriac will help gut flora to flourish, keeping that all important barrier function healthy. A velvety soup with deep roasted garlic flavour.

Ingredients

» 1 whole garlic bulb
» 1 tbsp olive oil
» 1 medium celeriac, peeled and diced
» 1 onion, chopped
» 700ml vegetable stock
» 200ml coconut milk
» Sea salt & black pepper, to taste
» Fresh thyme, to garnish

Method

» Preheat oven to 200°C (180°C fan). Slice the top off the garlic bulb, drizzle with olive oil, wrap in foil, and roast for 30 minutes.
» Heat olive oil in a saucepan, add the onion, and cook for 5 minutes.
» Add the celeriac and stock, then simmer for 20 minutes until tender.
» Squeeze the roasted garlic into the soup and blend until smooth.
» Stir in the coconut milk, season, and serve with fresh thyme.

Pumpkin & Red Lentil Soup

Smooth silky and satisfying. A hearty, protein-rich soup spiced with warming cumin and coriander. The lentils really help to make this low glycemic and feed your microbiome, not to mention keep you feeling full.

Ingredients

» 1 small pumpkin, peeled and diced (about 600g flesh)
» 1 onion, chopped
» 2 cloves garlic, minced
» 1-inch piece ginger, grated
» 100g red lentils, rinsed
» 800ml vegetable stock
» 1 tsp ground cumin
» ½ tsp ground coriander
» 200ml coconut milk
» 1 tbsp olive oil
» Sea salt & black pepper, to taste
» Fresh coriander, to serve

Method

» Heat olive oil in a saucepan, add onion, and cook for 5 minutes.
» Stir in garlic, ginger, cumin, and coriander. Cook for 1 minute.
» Add pumpkin, lentils, and stock. Simmer for 20 minutes until tender.
» Blend until smooth, then stir in coconut milk.
» Season and serve with fresh coriander.

Leek, Fennel & Salmon Chowder

A creamy, dairy-free chowder packed with the all important anti inflammatory long chain omega-3 fatty acids. A lighter fresher take on this classic.

Ingredients

- » 2 fillets salmon, skin removed, cut into chunks
- » 1 leek, finely sliced
- » 1 fennel bulb, thinly sliced
- » 2 cloves garlic, minced
- » 1 small potato, peeled and diced
- » 800ml fish or vegetable stock
- » 200ml coconut milk
- » 1 tbsp olive oil
- » Sea salt & black pepper, to taste
- » Fresh dill, to serve

Method

- » Heat olive oil in a saucepan, add leek and fennel, and cook for 5 minutes.
- » Stir in garlic and potato, then add stock. Simmer for 15 minutes.
- » Add the salmon and cook for 5 minutes.
- » Stir in coconut milk, season, and serve with fresh dill.

Broccoli, Kale & Almond Soup

A nutrient-dense soup rich in antioxidants and glucosinolates to support the production of ant-inflammatory chemicals and also keep our cells healthy. Winner

Ingredients

» 1 small broccoli, chopped into florets
» 50g kale, stems removed
» 1 onion, chopped
» 2 cloves garlic, minced
» 750ml vegetable stock
» 50g ground almonds
» 1 tbsp olive oil
» Sea salt & black pepper, to taste
» Flaked almonds, to serve

Method

» Heat olive oil in a saucepan, add the onion, and saute for 5 minutes.
» Add garlic, then broccoli, kale, and stock. Simmer for 10 minutes.
» Stir in ground almonds and blend until smooth.
» Season and serve with flaked almonds.

Mushroom & Thyme Soup

An earthy, umami-rich soup with a fragrant thyme finish. That combination of mushrooms and earthy herbs like thyme and rosemary is just heavenly. Especially in the winter.

Ingredients

» 250g chestnut mushrooms, sliced
» 1 onion, finely chopped
» 2 cloves garlic, minced
» 750ml vegetable stock
» 1 tsp fresh thyme leaves
» 200ml coconut milk
» 1 tbsp olive oil
» Sea salt & black pepper, to taste

Method

» Heat olive oil in a saucepan, add onion, and cook for 5 minutes.
» Stir in garlic and mushrooms, then cook for 10 minutes until softened.
» Add stock and thyme, then simmer for 10 minutes.
» Blend until smooth, stir in coconut milk, and season.

Cucumber & Avocado Chilled Soup

A refreshing, creamy cold soup perfect for warmer days. Can even be served as small shots as part of an al fresco dinner party. A nice hit of fatty acids, carotenoids and vitamin E to offer antioxidant protection.

Ingredients

» 1 large cucumber, peeled and chopped
» 1 ripe avocado, peeled and stoned
» 300ml cold vegetable stock
» 150g plain coconut yoghurt
» Juice of 1 lime
» 1 tbsp olive oil
» Sea salt & black pepper, to taste
» Fresh dill, to serve

Method

» This is a super easy one! Blend all ingredients until smooth.
» Chill for 30 minutes before serving.
» Garnish with fresh dill.

Curried Parsnip & Coconut Soup

Parsnips in a soup will always be a winner. The fact they have a powerful pre biotic activity that will help to nurture a healthy and diverse microbiome is just an added bonus.

Ingredients

» 3 medium parsnips, peeled and chopped
» 1 onion, chopped
» 2 cloves garlic, minced
» 1-inch piece ginger, grated
» 1 tsp mild curry powder
» 750ml vegetable stock
» 200ml coconut milk
» 1 tbsp olive oil
» Sea salt & black pepper, to taste
» Fresh coriander, to serve

Method

» Heat the olive oil and sauté the onion for about 5 minutes.
» Add the garlic, ginger, and curry powder. Cook for another minute.
» Add the parsnips and stock. Simmer for 20 minutes.
» Blend until smooth, stir in coconut milk, and season.

Pea & Mint Soup with Omega-3 Drizzle

A light, vibrant soup with a refreshing hint of mint. That age old combination works a dream. If there is any left over it can actually be great as a sauce too!

Ingredients

» 400g frozen peas
» 1 small onion, chopped
» 750ml vegetable stock
» 2 tbsp fresh mint, chopped
» 1 tbsp olive oil
» 1 tbsp flaxseed oil, for drizzling
» Sea salt & black pepper, to taste

Method

» Sauté the onion in olive oil for 5 minutes or so.
» Add the peas and stock. Simmer for 5 minutes.
» Blend with mint until smooth.
» Drizzle with flaxseed oil before serving.

Spicy Roasted Tomato & Basil Soup

A classic made even better. Carotenoid rich tomatoes provide a beautiful bath of antioxidant activity. A rich, oven-roasted tomato soup with a hint of spice.

Ingredients

- » 800g ripe tomatoes, halved
- » 1 onion, quartered
- » 3 cloves garlic, whole
- » 1 tbsp olive oil
- » 750ml vegetable stock
- » ½ tsp chilli flakes
- » 2 tbsp fresh basil, chopped
- » Sea salt & black pepper, to taste

Method

- » Preheat the oven to 200°C (180°C fan).
- » Place the tomatoes, onion, and garlic on a tray. Drizzle with olive oil and roast for 30 minutes.
- » Transfer to a saucepan, add stock and chilli flakes. Simmer for 5 minutes.
- » Blend until smooth, stir in basil, and season.

Asparagus & Lemon Soup

A squeeze of lemon over lightly cooked asparagus is an absolute dream with a weekend breakfast. So, why would that combo not work perfectly well in a soup?

Ingredients

- » 1 bunch asparagus, trimmed and chopped
- » 1 onion, chopped
- » 2 cloves garlic, minced
- » 750ml vegetable stock
- » Juice of 1 lemon
- » 1 tbsp olive oil
- » Sea salt & black pepper, to taste
- » Flaked almonds, to serve

Method

- » In a little olive oil, sauté the onion and garlic for around 5 mins, until the onion has softened.
- » Add the asparagus and stock. Simmer for 10 minutes.
- » Blend until smooth, stir in lemon juice, and season.
- » Garnish with flaked almonds.

Beetroot & Ginger Soup

Beetroot in a soup is just a powerful thing. Flavour wise. Colour wise and health benefit wise too. If you wanted to add an extra spicy dimension to this, you could garnish it with dollop of horseradish sauce.

Ingredients

- » 3 medium beetroots, peeled and chopped
- » 1 onion, chopped
- » 2 cloves garlic, minced
- » 1-inch piece ginger, grated
- » 750ml vegetable stock
- » 1 tbsp olive oil
- » Sea salt & black pepper, to taste
- » Coconut yoghurt, to serve

Method

- » Heat olive oil and sauté the onion, garlic, and ginger for 5 minutes. ideally you want the onion to be soft and translucent.
- » Add the beetroots and enough stock to covers. Simmer for 25 minutes.
- » Once the beetroot has softened, blend until smooth, season, and serve with a dollop of coconut yoghurt.

Butternut Squash & Sage Soup

This is a classic combo. Butternut squash and sage really are a flavour match made in heaven.

Ingredients

» 1 small butternut squash, peeled and diced
» 1 red onion, chopped
» 2 cloves garlic, minced
» 750ml vegetable stock

» 1 tbsp fresh sage, chopped
» 1 tbsp olive oil
» Sea salt & black pepper, to taste

Method

» Sauté the onion and garlic in a little olive oil, along with a good pinch of sea salt until the onion softens.
» Add the sage and sauté for another 2-3 minutes.
» Add the diced squash, and enough stock to cover. Simmer until the squash softens.
» Once the squash is soft, blend until smooth and season.

Courgette & Dill Soup

A light, summery soup with fresh dill. Doesn't get much easier.

Ingredients

- » 2 large courgettes, chopped
- » 1 onion, chopped
- » 2 cloves garlic, minced
- » 750ml vegetable stock
- » 1 tbsp fresh dill, chopped
- » 1 tbsp olive oil
- » Sea salt & black pepper, to taste

Method

- » Heat the olive oil and sauté the onion and garlic for 5 minutes.
- » Add the courgettes and stock. Simmer for 10 minutes.
- » Blend until smooth, stir in dill, and season.

Red Cabbage & Apple Slaw (Starter Salad)

A crispy crunchy polyphenol powerhouse. Raw red cabbage marries so perfectly with apple. There is sweetness. Spiciness. Juiciness. Crunchiness. What a winner.

Ingredients

» ½ red cabbage - finely shredded
» 1 apple - julienned
» 1 tbsp flaxseed oil
» 1 tbsp apple cider vinegar
» 1 tsp Dijon mustard
» Sea salt & black pepper, to taste
» Walnuts, chopped, to serve

Method

» Toss the shredded cabbage and julienned apple into a bowl.
» Whisk together the flaxseed oil, vinegar, mustard, salt, and pepper until fully combined.
» Drizzle over the slaw, mix well, and top with walnuts.

LUNCHES

If there is one area that really does trip people up, it is lunches throughout the working week. If you don't get organised and have good stuff on hand and have an array of recipes that you can easily prepare that meet your goals, then it is all too easy to go to the fast food outlets or opt for a pub lunch. These recipes can be great made ahead for on the go, or are a perfect option for a leisurely lunch at home.

Salmon & Avocado Wraps

A fresh, omega-3-rich alternative to traditional wraps. The crunch you get from the lettuce is a nice contrast. You can of course use bread wraps if you want to, just remember the golden rule - make sure they are whole wheat or multigrain versions. Keep the white ones off your table

Ingredients

» 2 ripe avocados, sliced
» 2 fillets cooked salmon, flaked
» 8 large romaine or cos lettuce leaves
» 1 red pepper, sliced
» ½ cucumber, sliced
» 50g of feta cheese
» Juice of 1 lemon
» 1 tbsp extra virgin olive oil
» Sea salt & black pepper, to taste

Method

» Lay out the lettuce leaves as wraps.
» Evenly distribute the salmon, avocado, red pepper, and cucumber.
» Crumble in the feta cheese.
» Drizzle with lemon juice and olive oil.
» Season, wrap, and serve immediately.

Mackerel Pâté with Crudités

A creamy, omega-3-packed pâté with a zesty kick. This is a bit of a classic this one. Great with chunks of radish, carrot sticks, even wedges of raw red cabbage.

Ingredients

- » 2 fillets smoked mackerel, skin removed
- » 100g plain coconut yoghurt
- » Juice of 1 lemon
- » 1 tbsp fresh dill, chopped
- » Sea salt & black pepper, to taste
- » 1 carrot, sliced into sticks
- » 1 red pepper, sliced
- » ½ cucumber, sliced

Method

- » Flake the mackerel into a blender or food processor. Add the yoghurt, lemon juice, and dill and then blend until smooth.
- » Season to taste.
- » Serve with the vegetable crudités.

Spinach & Walnut Pesto Courgetti

Ok, I am going to go there. I know that this is usually the territory of the trendy online influencers - courgetti. Making spaghetti out of courgettes using a spiraliser or vegetable peeler. Forget the trendiness. These are actually a great option if you want that spaghetti vibe but want to reign the carbs in a little.

Ingredients

» 2 large or 4 small courgettes (zucchini's)
» 60g walnuts
» 100g spinach
» 1 clove garlic, minced
» 2tbsp of grated parmesan cheese
» Juice of 1 lemon
» 3 tbsp extra virgin olive oil
» Sea salt & black pepper, to taste

Method

» Start off by turning the courgettes into noodles. You can of course use a spiraliser - one of those twisty gadgets that turn veg into perfect spaghetti type noodles. Or, for an easier way to do things, make flat noodles by running a vegetable peeler along the body of the courgette to make thin flat ribbon type noodles. Whichever you prefer.
» Blend the walnuts, spinach, garlic, lemon juice, parmesan and olive oil into a pesto. Play around with the texture and add a little more olive oil if you want to.
» Toss with the courgetti and season before serving.

Tuna & Olive Salad with Flax Yogurt Dressing

Who doesn't love a good tuna salad? It doesn't have to be that boring old school staple. We can jazz it up a bit. Tuna is a great source of EPA & DHA, Zinc and selenium. Bonus! A simple but nutrient-dense salad with a Mediterranean twist.

Ingredients

» 2 tins tuna in olive oil, drained
» 100g black olives, sliced
» 1 red onion, finely sliced
» 1 cucumber, diced
» 1 heaped tbsp of plain yogurt
» 1 tsp of Dijon mustard
» 1 tbsp flaxseed oil
» Juice of 1 lemon
» Sea salt & black pepper, to taste

Method

» Toss the tuna, onions, olives and cucumber together in a large bowl.
» Add the dijon, the yogurt, flax oil and lemon juice together and whisk well with a fork to make a smooth dressing.
» Pour this all over the tuna mix and stir it all together.
» Season and serve.

Chickpea & Red Pepper Hummus Bowl

I am a self confessed hummusholic. I absolutely love the stuff. The red peppers in this dish give us some anti-inflammatory polyphenols and the diversity of fibre is a party for our microbiome. A protein-packed, fibre-rich dish.

Ingredients

» 1 tin chickpeas, drained
» 1 red pepper - sliced and deseeded
» 1 tbsp tahini
» Juice of 1 lemon
» 1 clove garlic, minced
» 1 tbsp extra virgin olive oil
» Sea salt & black pepper, to taste
» Cucumber & radish slices, to serve

Method

» Pre heat the oven to 180.
» Place the sliced peppers into a roasting tin and drizzle with olive oil. Roast for around 20 minutes until the pepper is soft.
» Add the chickpeas, roasted pepper, tahini, lemon juice, garlic, and olive oil into a blender and blitz into a smooth hummus.
» Serve with cucumber and radish slices.

Grilled Sardine & Fennel Salad

This is a real omega 3 dense powerhouse of a dish. Sardines are hands down one of the best sources of the potently anti-inflammatory long chain omega 3 fatty acids EPA & DHA. This is a light and refreshing salad with a serious boost.

Ingredients

» 4 cooked sardines
» 1 fennel bulb
» 1 orange, segmented

» 1 tbsp extra virgin olive oil
» Sea salt & black pepper, to taste

Method

» Flake the cooked sardines with a fork. Remove any large bones. The small ones are perfectly fine and can be a good source of calcium, but if you struggle to chew or if you choke easily, then pull them all out. Flake the fish well.
» Thinly slice the fennel.
» Gently toss all the ingredients together in a large bowl.
» Drizzle with olive oil and season before serving.

Spiced Lentil & Beetroot Salad

I have done so many variations of this dish over the years. The marriage of beetroot and lentil is a perfect one. Whether it is cooked beetroot cut into wedges, or like this one, some raw beetroot. It just blends perfectly.

Ingredients

» 200g puy lentils - from the tine. Drained.
» 2 medium raw beetroot
» 80g feta cheese
» 1 tbsp extra virgin olive oil
» 1 tsp ground cumin
» Juice of 1 lemon
» Sea salt & black pepper, to taste
» Fresh coriander, to garnish

Method

» Grate the beetroot into a bowl (you may want to wear gloves for that one).
» Add the cooked lentils and crumble in the feta cheese.
» Add the olive oil, lemon juice, cumin and the salt & pepper to taste.
» Serve garnished with fresh coriander.

Roasted Broccoli & Almond Salad

Ok this sounds a bit drab I know, but when you roast broccoli, something magical happens. The texture of the floret edges are just heavenly. A vibrant, crunchy, antioxidant-rich dish.

Ingredients

» 1 **head broccoli**, cut into florets
» 30g **almonds**, chopped
» 1 tbsp **extra virgin olive oil**
» Juice of **1 lemon**
» **Sea salt & black pepper**, to taste

Method

» Pre heat oven to 200.
» Drizzle the broccoli florets with a little olive oil and a pinch of salt, and spread on a baking tray.
» Roast for 20-25 minutes until soft and turning golden at the edges. That is where the magic happens.
» Toss with almonds and lemon juice.

Celeriac Remoulade with Smoked Trout

This beautiful lighter version of a remoulade packs a beautiful flavour and keeps for a few days in the fridge too. That marriage of the earthy celeriac ad the smokey trout is just perfect. A crunchy, creamy dish with a punchy dressing.

Ingredients

» 1 small celeriac
» 100g plain coconut yoghurt
» Juice of 1 lemon
» 1 tsp Dijon mustard

» 2 fillets smoked trout, flaked
» Sea salt & black pepper, to taste

Method

» Grate the celeriac and then mix with the yoghurt, lemon juice, and mustard.
» Top with smoked trout and season.

Curried Cauliflower & Lentil Salad

Cauliflower is another one of those vegetables that comes alive in new ways when you roast it and give it a lovely crispy edge. Normally I thoroughly dislike cauliflower. Roast it, a whole different story. A protein-rich, spiced salad with warming flavours.

Ingredients

» 1 small cauliflower, cut into florets
» 1 tbsp olive oil
» 1 tsp ground cumin
» 1 tsp turmeric
» 200g puy lentils, cooked
» 1 small red onion, finely sliced
» Juice of 1 lemon
» 1 tbsp extra virgin olive oil
» Sea salt & black pepper, to taste
» Fresh coriander, to garnish

Method

» Preheat oven to 200°C (180°C fan). Toss cauliflower with olive oil, cumin, and turmeric.
» Roast for 25 minutes until golden and tender.
» Mix with cooked lentils, red onion, lemon juice, and extra olive oil.
» Season and garnish with coriander.

Grilled Aubergine with Walnut Salsa

Aubergines do love a smokey flavour. It matches so beautifully. A simple, nutrient-dense dish with a garlicky walnut topping.

Ingredients

» 2 large aubergines, halved
» Half a teaspoon of smoked paprika
» 1 tbsp olive oil
» 50g walnuts, finely chopped
» 1 clove garlic, minced
» 1 tbsp extra virgin olive oil
» Juice of 1 lemon
» 1 tbsp fresh parsley, chopped
» Sea salt & black pepper, to taste

Method

» Preheat oven to 200°C (180°C fan).
» Brush aubergines with olive oil and roast for 30 minutes.
» Mix walnuts, garlic, extra virgin olive oil, lemon juice, and parsley.
» Spoon walnut salsa over the grilled aubergines and serve.

Courgette Fritters with Tzatziki

I do love a courgette fritter. Best served overlooking the Mediterranean sea, but if that isn't an option, then your kitchen table will do. A low-carb, crispy fritter served with a cooling yoghurt dip.

Ingredients

» *For the fritters:*
» 2 large courgettes, grated
» 1 egg, beaten
» 50g ground almonds
» 1 tsp cumin
» 1 tbsp olive oil
» Sea salt & black pepper, to taste

» *For the tzatziki:*
» 150g plain coconut yoghurt
» ½ cucumber, grated
» 1 clove garlic, minced
» 1 tbsp fresh mint, chopped
» Juice of ½ lemon

Method

» Place grated courgette in a clean tea towel and squeeze out excess water.
» Mix courgette with egg, ground almonds, cumin, salt, and pepper.
» Shape into fritters and fry in olive oil over medium heat until golden.
» For tzatziki, mix all ingredients together in a bowl.
» Serve fritters with a dollop of tzatziki.

Stuffed Peppers with Quinoa & Herbs

A protein-rich, plant-based meal with a delicious flavour profile. The sweetness of the peppers is matched beautifully with the sharp tang of the feta.

Ingredients

»   4 large bell peppers, halved and deseeded
»   200g quinoa, cooked
»   1 small red onion, finely chopped
»   2 cloves garlic, minced
»   7-8 black olives - roughly chopped
»   1 tbsp olive oil
»   1 tsp ground cumin
»   1 tbsp fresh parsley, chopped
»   1 tbsp fresh coriander, chopped
»   80g Feta Cheese
»   Sea salt & black pepper, to taste

Method

»   Preheat oven to 200°C (180°C fan).
»   Heat olive oil in a pan and sauté onion and garlic for 5 minutes.
»   Stir in cooked quinoa, cumin, parsley, olives and coriander. Season to taste.
»   Fill the pepper halves with the quinoa mixture.
»   Bake for 25 minutes until the peppers are tender.
»   Crumble over the feta and return to the oven for 5 minutes.

Mushroom & Spinach Omelette

Omelettes aren't just for breakfast you know. The only pointer I will give here is if you had eggs for breakfast, don't have them for lunch. Vary things as much as you can. A simple yet nutrient-dense lunch option.

Ingredients

» 6 eggs, beaten
» 200g chestnut mushrooms, sliced
» 100g spinach, chopped
» 1 tbsp olive oil
» Sea salt & black pepper, to taste

Method

» Heat olive oil in a frying pan. Sauté mushrooms for 5 minutes.
» Add spinach and cook for another minute.
» Pour in beaten eggs, season, and cook until set.
» Fold and serve immediately.

So many people find that they come unstuck at dinner time. After a long day you want something that feeds the soul as much as it feeds the body. It can be really tempting to reach for unhealthy comfort foods. Another problem is that different family members may not be on your healthy eating path. However, if you can create recipes that taste absolutely heavenly and are family friendly, and that

Baked Salmon with Walnut & Herb Crust

A crispy, omega-3-rich salmon dish with a fragrant nutty crust. This is a great one to pull out at a dinner party or for a Friday night feast.

Ingredients

- » 4 fillets salmon (about 150g each)
- » 60g walnuts, finely chopped
- » 1 tbsp fresh parsley, finely chopped
- » 1 tbsp fresh thyme, finely chopped
- » 1 clove garlic, minced
- » 1 tbsp extra virgin olive oil
- » 1 tsp Dijon mustard
- » Zest of 1 lemon
- » Juice of ½ lemon
- » Sea salt & black pepper, to taste

Method

- » Preheat the oven to 200°C (180°C fan). Line a baking tray with parchment paper.
- » In a small bowl, mix the walnuts, parsley, thyme, garlic, olive oil, mustard, lemon zest, and juice.
- » Season with salt and pepper.
- » Place the salmon fillets on the baking tray, skin-side down. Press the walnut mixture firmly on top of each fillet to create an even crust.

» Bake for 12-15 minutes or until the salmon is cooked through and the crust is golden.
» Serve immediately with steamed greens or a light salad.

Roast Chicken with Lemon & Thyme

One of my absolute favourite things to cook is a roast. I love the theatre of it. This is a perfect centre piece for one. Served with some sweet potato wedges and lightly cooked greens it is perfect.

Ingredients

- » 1 whole free-range chicken (about 1.5kg)
- » 2 tbsp extra virgin olive oil
- » 1 lemon, halved
- » 4 sprigs fresh thyme
- » 4 cloves garlic, crushed
- » 1 tsp turmeric
- » Sea salt & black pepper, to taste

Method

- » Preheat the oven to 200°C (180°C fan).
- » Pat the chicken dry with kitchen paper. Rub the skin with olive oil, turmeric, salt, and pepper.
- » Stuff the cavity with the lemon halves, thyme, and crushed garlic.
- » Place the chicken on a roasting tray, breast-side up. Roast for 1 hour 20 minutes, basting with the juices halfway through.
- » To check doneness, insert a skewer into the thickest part of the thigh; the juices should run clear.
- » Rest for 15 minutes before carving. Serve with roasted vegetables or a fresh green salad.

Braised Lamb Shoulder with Garlic & Rosemary

A melt-in-the-mouth, slow-cooked lamb dish with deep, aromatic flavours. Another great family friendly centre piece.

Ingredients

» 1kg lamb shoulder, bone-in
» 1 tbsp extra virgin olive oil
» 4 cloves garlic, sliced
» 2 sprigs rosemary, leaves removed

» 1 tsp ground cumin
» 500ml beef or lamb stock
» 1 tbsp apple cider vinegar
» Sea salt & black pepper, to taste

Method

» Preheat oven to 160°C (140°C fan).
» Heat the olive oil in a large ovenproof casserole dish. Sear the lamb shoulder for 3-4 minutes per side until browned.
» Remove the lamb and set aside. In the same dish, add garlic and rosemary, cooking for 1 minute.
» Return the lamb to the dish, sprinkle with cumin, then pour in the stock and vinegar.
» Cover with a lid and transfer to the oven. Cook for 3-4 hours, basting occasionally, until the meat is tender and falling off the bone.
» Serve with roasted root vegetables or steamed greens.

Spicy Turkey & Spinach Meatballs

A lean, protein-rich meal with a bold, spiced tomato sauce to pack an anti-inflammatory punch.

Ingredients

» *For the meatballs:*
» 400g turkey mince
» 1 onion, finely grated
» 1 clove garlic, minced
» 1 tsp ground cumin
» 1 tsp smoked paprika
» 1 tbsp fresh parsley, chopped
» Sea salt & black pepper, to taste

» *For the sauce:*
» 1 tin chopped tomatoes
» 1 tbsp tomato purée
» 1 clove garlic, minced
» 100g fresh spinach, chopped
» 1 tsp ground turmeric
» 1 tbsp extra virgin olive oil

Method

» Preheat oven to 200°C (180°C fan).
» In a bowl, mix all the meatball ingredients. Shape into small balls and place on a lined baking tray.
» Bake for 15 minutes until golden.
» Meanwhile, heat olive oil in a pan, add garlic, then stir in the tomatoes, tomato purée, turmeric, and spinach. Simmer for 10 minutes.
» Add the meatballs to the sauce and simmer for 5 more minutes.
» Serve with steamed greens or cauliflower rice.

Lentil & Aubergine Moussaka

I have done so many versions of this dish over the years and it is always a crowd pleaser. Fibre rich to feed the microbiome and packed with anti-inflammatory phytochemicals. A rich, layered Mediterranean-inspired dish without dairy or refined carbohydrates. You can of course do a dairy version if you wanted by combining yogurt, eggs and feta cheese as the topping.

Ingredients

» *For the lentil filling:*
» 200g puy lentils, cooked
» 1 onion, finely chopped
» 2 cloves garlic, minced
» 1 tin chopped tomatoes
» 1 tbsp tomato purée
» 1 tsp ground cinnamon
» 1 tsp dried oregano
» 1 tbsp extra virgin olive oil
» Sea salt & black pepper, to taste

» *For the aubergines:*
» 2 large aubergines, sliced into rounds
» 1 tbsp extra virgin olive oil
» *For the cashew topping:*
» 100g cashews, soaked in boiling water for 15 minutes
» 1 tbsp nutritional yeast
» Juice of ½ lemon
» 100ml coconut milk

Method

» Preheat oven to 200°C (180°C fan).
» Heat olive oil in a saucepan. Sauté onion and garlic for 5 minutes. Add the lentils, chopped tomatoes, tomato purée, cinnamon, oregano, salt, and pepper. Simmer for 10 minutes.
» Meanwhile, brush aubergine slices with olive oil and grill for 4 minutes per side until golden.
» Blend the cashews, nutritional yeast, lemon juice, and coconut milk into a creamy sauce.
» In a baking dish, layer half the aubergines, then the lentil mixture, then the remaining aubergines. Pour the cashew sauce over the top.
» Bake for 20 minutes until golden. Let rest for 5 minutes before serving.

Stuffed Butternut Squash with Quinoa & Pumpkin Seeds

A hearty, vibrant plant-based meal packed with fibre and nutrients. The orange colour of the butternut squash is the key anti-inflammatory power nutrient here.

Ingredients

» 1 butternut squash, halved lengthways and deseeded
» 1 tbsp olive oil
» 200g quinoa, cooked
» 1 small red onion, finely chopped
» 1 clove garlic, minced
» 1 tsp ground cumin
» 50g pumpkin seeds
» 1 tbsp fresh coriander, chopped
» Sea salt & black pepper, to taste

Method

» Preheat oven to 200°C (180°C fan). Brush squash halves with olive oil and season. Place cut-side up on a baking tray and roast for 40 minutes until soft.
» Meanwhile, heat olive oil in a pan. Sauté onion and garlic for 5 minutes. Add cumin, cooked quinoa, and pumpkin seeds. Stir well and cook for 2 more minutes.
» Scoop out some of the squash flesh to create a cavity, then mix it into the quinoa filling.
» Stuff the mixture back into the squash halves and bake for another 10 minutes. Garnish with fresh coriander before serving.

Cod with Puy Lentils & Mustard Dressing

To me this is a perfect dinner. High protein, high fibre and a bucket full of flavour. A simple yet elegant dish with a rich, tangy dressing.

Ingredients

» 4 fillets cod (about 150g each)
» 200g puy lentils, cooked
» 1 red onion, finely chopped
» 1 tbsp extra virgin olive oil
» 1 tbsp Dijon mustard
» Juice of 1 lemon
» 1 tbsp fresh parsley, chopped
» Sea salt & black pepper, to taste

Method

» Preheat oven to 200°C (180°C fan). Place the cod fillets on a lined baking tray, season, and bake for 12-15 minutes.
» Heat olive oil in a pan and sauté the red onion for 5 minutes. Stir in the cooked lentils, mustard, lemon juice, salt, and pepper.
» Serve the cod on a bed of lentils, garnished with fresh parsley.

Beef & Cabbage Stir-Fry

This is the kind of thing that I often whip up in the evenings at home. A quick and flavourful stir-fry. You can substitute the coconut aminos for soy sauce.

Ingredients

» 400g beef sirloin, thinly sliced
» ½ green cabbage, shredded
» 1 carrot, julienned
» 1 red pepper, sliced
» 2 cloves garlic, minced
» 1-inch piece ginger, grated
» 1 tbsp coconut aminos
» 1 tbsp extra virgin olive oil
» Sea salt & black pepper, to taste

Method

» Heat olive oil in a wok over high heat. Add beef and sear for 2-3 minutes, then remove and set aside.
» In the same pan, sauté garlic and ginger for 30 seconds. Add cabbage, carrot, and red pepper. Stir-fry for 3-4 minutes.
» Return the beef to the pan, add coconut aminos, and cook for 1 more minute.
» Serve immediately.

Baked Trout with Caper & Dill Butter

Trout is such a delicious fish, yet always seems to take a back-seat to salmon. Give it a try more often. A light and flavourful dish with a zesty butter sauce.

Ingredients

» 4 fillets trout
» 1 tbsp olive oil
» Juice of 1 lemon
» 1 tbsp capers, drained and chopped

» 1 tbsp fresh dill, chopped
» Sea salt & black pepper, to taste

Method

» Preheat oven to 200°C (180°C fan). Brush trout fillets with olive oil and season.
» Place on a baking tray and bake for 12 minutes.
» Meanwhile, mix lemon juice, capers, and dill in a small bowl.
» Spoon the dressing over the trout and serve immediately.

Turmeric-Spiced Chicken & Cauliflower Rice

I have drummed it in that we need to opt for a low glycemic diet. This does not mean giving up carbohydrates completely, but part of it certainly is reigning them in a little. Cauliflower rice is a great way to do that.

Ingredients

» 4 chicken breasts, sliced
» 1 tbsp extra virgin olive oil
» 1 tsp turmeric
» 1 tsp ground cumin
» 1 clove garlic, minced
» 1 cauliflower, grated into rice
» Juice of 1 lemon
» Sea salt & black pepper, to taste

Method

» Heat olive oil in a frying pan. Toss the chicken with turmeric, cumin, garlic, salt, and pepper.
» Cook the chicken for 8-10 minutes, turning halfway, until golden and cooked through.
» In a separate pan, heat a little oil and sauté the cauliflower rice for 2-3 minutes.
» Serve the chicken over the cauliflower rice, drizzled with lemon juice.

Grilled Lamb Chops with Mint & Garlic

Tender lamb chops infused with fresh mint and garlic, served with courgettes. A classic combination and a long term favourite.

Ingredients

» 8 lamb chops
» 2 cloves garlic, minced
» 1 tbsp fresh mint, chopped
» Juice of 1 lemon
» 1 tbsp extra virgin olive oil
» Sea salt & black pepper, to taste
» 2 medium courgettes, sliced into rounds

Method

» In a bowl, mix garlic, mint, lemon juice, olive oil, salt, and pepper.
» Coat the lamb chops with the marinade and let sit for 30 minutes.
» Preheat a grill or griddle pan to medium-high heat.
» Grill the lamb chops for 3-4 minutes per side for medium-rare or longer for well done.
» Meanwhile, grill the courgette slices for 2 minutes per side.
» Serve the lamb with the grilled courgettes.

Sweet Potato & Chickpea Coconut Curry

A fragrant, creamy curry spiced with turmeric and ginger. I absolutely adore this combination and I think you will find that it soon becomes a family favourite.

Ingredients

- 2 medium sweet potatoes, peeled and diced
- 1 tin chickpeas, drained
- 1 onion, chopped
- 2 cloves garlic, minced
- 1-inch piece ginger, grated
- 1 tsp turmeric
- 1 tsp ground coriander
- 1 tsp ground cumin
- 1 tin coconut milk
- 400ml vegetable stock
- 1 tbsp extra virgin olive oil
- Sea salt & black pepper, to taste
- 1 tbsp fresh coriander, chopped

Method

- Heat olive oil in a large pan. Sauté onion, garlic, and ginger for 5 minutes.
- Stir in turmeric, coriander, and cumin. Cook for 1 minute to release flavours.
- Add sweet potatoes, chickpeas, coconut milk, and stock. Simmer for 20 minutes, stirring occasionally.
- Check seasoning and adjust as needed.
- Serve garnished with fresh coriander.

Rosemary & Garlic Roasted Duck Breast

A rich, flavourful dish with crispy skin and aromatic herbs.

Ingredients

- 4 duck breasts, skin scored
- 2 sprigs rosemary, leaves chopped
- 2 cloves garlic, minced
- Sea salt & black pepper, to taste

Method

- Preheat oven to 200°C (180°C fan).
- Rub the duck breasts with rosemary, garlic, salt, and pepper.
- Place the duck skin-side down in a cold pan over medium heat. Cook for 6-7 minutes until the skin is crisp and golden.
- Flip the duck and sear for 1 minute on the other side.
- Transfer to the oven and roast for 6-8 minutes for medium.
- Rest for 5 minutes before slicing and serving.
- Perfect with. a pea puree or buttered greens

Slow-Cooked Beef & Mushroom Stew

This is true comfort food and a perfect winter warmer. A warming, deeply flavoured dish perfect for slow cooking.

Ingredients

» 600g beef stewing steak, cubed
» 200g chestnut mushrooms, sliced
» 1 onion, chopped
» 2 cloves garlic, minced
» 750ml beef stock
» 1 tbsp tomato purée
» 1 tsp fresh thyme, chopped
» 1 tbsp extra virgin olive oil
» Sea salt & black pepper, to taste

Method

» Heat olive oil in a large pan. Brown the beef in batches, then set aside.
» In the same pan, sauté onion and garlic for 5 minutes.
» Stir in mushrooms and cook for 3 minutes.
» Add tomato purée, thyme, and stock. Bring to a simmer.
» Return the beef to the pan, cover, and cook on low heat for 2½-3 hours, stirring occasionally, until the beef is tender.
» Serve hot with steamed greens and mashed celeriac.

Cod & Spinach Coconut Curry

White fish like cod works beautifully in a curry, but do stir it gently as it will quickly fall apart. A delicate, mild fish curry infused with coconut and turmeric.

Ingredients

- » 4 fillets cod
- » 200g fresh spinach
- » 1 onion, chopped
- » 2 cloves garlic, minced
- » 1-inch piece ginger, grated
- » 1 tsp turmeric
- » 1 tin coconut milk
- » 400ml fish stock
- » 1 tbsp extra virgin olive oil
- » Sea salt & black pepper, to taste
- » 1 tbsp fresh coriander, chopped

Method

- » Heat olive oil in a pan. Sauté onion, garlic, and ginger for 5 minutes.
- » Stir in turmeric, then pour in coconut milk and fish stock. Simmer for 5 minutes.
- » Add cod fillets and gently poach for 8 minutes, or until cooked through.
- » Stir in fresh spinach and cook for 1 minute until wilted.
- » Serve garnished with coriander.

SIDES

With all of these great lunches and dinners, you will need something just as powerful and delicious to serve along side them. This section has you covered.

Roasted Brussels Sprouts with Walnuts & Lemon

I am absolutely obsessed with roasted sprouts. I have them a couple of times a week. If you have never tried a roasted sprout, then do yourself a favour and give them a bash. A crunchy, nutty side dish with a bright citrus finish.

Ingredients

» 500g Brussels sprouts, trimmed and halved
» 1 tbsp extra virgin olive oil
» 50g walnuts, roughly chopped
» Zest of 1 lemon
» Juice of ½ lemon
» Sea salt & black pepper, to taste

Method

» Preheat the oven to 200°C (180°C fan).
» Toss the Brussels sprouts with olive oil, salt, and pepper on a baking tray. Spread them out in a single layer.
» Roast for 20-25 minutes, stirring halfway, until golden and crispy.
» In the last 5 minutes, scatter the walnuts onto the tray to toast them.
» Remove from the oven, drizzle with lemon juice, and toss with the lemon zest.
» Serve warm.

Garlic & Chilli Kale Chips

These could easily be a snack or a side. You pick! Crispy, flavour-packed kale chips with a spicy kick.

Ingredients

» 200g kale, stems removed and leaves torn
» 1 tbsp extra virgin olive oil
» 1 clove garlic, finely grated
» ½ tsp chilli flakes
» Sea salt, to taste

Method

» Preheat the oven to 150°C (130°C fan).
» Massage the kale with olive oil, garlic, chilli flakes, and salt.
» Spread out on a baking tray in a single layer.
» Bake for 12-15 minutes, checking regularly, until crisp but not burnt.
» Serve immediately.

Turmeric-Spiced Roasted Cauliflower

This is a perfect side for fish or roasted meats, or on their own with a bowl of hummus.

Ingredients

» 1 medium cauliflower, cut into florets
» 1 tbsp extra virgin olive oil
» 1 tsp turmeric
» ½ tsp ground cumin
» ½ tsp ground coriander
» Sea salt & black pepper, to taste

Method

» Preheat the oven to 200°C (180°C fan).
» Toss cauliflower with olive oil, turmeric, cumin, coriander, salt, and pepper.
» Spread onto a lined baking tray and roast for 20-25 minutes, stirring halfway, until golden.
» Serve hot.

Courgette & Walnut Slaw

A light, refreshing slaw with a nutty crunch. This will work perfectly alongside a light alfresco lunch.

Ingredients

» 2 large courgettes, grated
» 50g walnuts, chopped
» 1 tbsp extra virgin olive oil
» Juice of ½ lemon
» Sea salt & black pepper, to taste

Method

» Place grated courgettes in a clean tea towel and squeeze out excess water.
» Toss courgettes with walnuts, olive oil, lemon juice, salt, and pepper.
» Serve immediately.

Celeriac & Garlic Mash

A creamy, low-carb alternative to mashed potatoes.

Ingredients

» 1 medium celeriac, peeled and diced
» 2 cloves garlic, peeled
» 200ml coconut milk
» 1 tbsp extra virgin olive oil
» Sea salt & black pepper, to taste

Method

» Boil celeriac and garlic in salted water for 15-20 minutes, until soft.
» Drain, then mash with coconut milk, olive oil, salt, and pepper.
» Serve warm.

Beetroot & Dill Pickled Slaw

This flavour combination works beautifully. A tangy, probiotic-rich side dish.

Ingredients

» 2 medium beetroots, grated
» ½ red onion, finely sliced
» 2 tbsp apple cider vinegar
» 1 tbsp extra virgin olive oil
» 1 tbsp fresh dill, chopped
» Sea salt & black pepper, to taste

Method

» Toss all ingredients together in a bowl.
» Let sit for 10 minutes before serving.

Roasted Butternut Squash with Thyme

A simple, flavourful roasted vegetable side. Great with roasted meats or incorporated into a salad.

Ingredients

» 1 small butternut squash, peeled and cubed
» 1 tbsp extra virgin olive oil
» 1 tbsp fresh thyme
» Sea salt & black pepper, to taste

Method

» Preheat oven to 200°C (180°C fan).
» Toss butternut squash with olive oil, thyme, salt, and pepper.
» Roast for 30 minutes, stirring halfway, until tender and caramelised.

Miso & Sesame Roasted Aubergine

Hands down this has to be one of my favourite things on the planet. Miso aubergine is just mind blowing. Give it a try and you will see what I mean. A deep, umami-rich side with white miso.

Ingredients

» 2 large aubergines, halved
» 1 tbsp white miso paste
» 1 tbsp extra virgin olive oil

» 1 tsp toasted sesame seeds
» Sea salt, to taste

Method

» Preheat oven to 200°C (180°C fan).
» Mix miso and olive oil, then brush onto aubergine halves.
» Roast for 25-30 minutes until soft and golden.
» Sprinkle with sesame seeds before serving.

Roasted Carrots with Cumin & Coriander

A spiced take on roasted carrots. Cumin blends with carrot so perfectly.

Ingredients

» 4 medium carrots, cut into batons
» 1 tbsp extra virgin olive oil
» ½ tsp ground cumin
» ½ tsp ground coriander
» Sea salt & black pepper, to taste

Method

» Preheat oven to 200°C (180°C fan).
» Toss carrots with olive oil, cumin, coriander, salt, and pepper.
» Roast for 25 minutes, stirring halfway.

Avocado & Flaxseed Dressing

A creamy, nutrient-dense sauce for drizzling or dipping.

Ingredients

- » 1 ripe avocado
- » 1 tbsp flaxseed oil
- » Juice of 1 lemon
- » Sea salt & black pepper, to taste

Method

- » Blend all ingredients until smooth.
- » Adjust consistency with water if needed.

Spinach & Lemon Sauté

A light and zesty side dish that enhances the natural flavour of spinach.

Ingredients

» 200g fresh spinach
» 1 tbsp extra virgin olive oil
» Juice of ½ lemon
» 1 clove garlic, minced
» Sea salt & black pepper, to taste

Method

» Heat the olive oil in a large pan over medium heat.
» Add the garlic and cook for 30 seconds until fragrant.
» Add the spinach and stir continuously for 2-3 minutes until wilted.
» Remove from heat, drizzle with lemon juice, and season with salt and pepper.
» Serve immediately.

Grilled Asparagus with Garlic Butter

A simple yet flavourful side that pairs well with fish or poultry. I also love this at breakfast time with a couple of poached eggs.

Ingredients

» 1 bunch asparagus, trimmed
» 1 tbsp extra virgin olive oil
» 1 clove garlic, minced
» 1 tbsp unsalted butter (or coconut oil for dairy-free)
» Sea salt & black pepper, to taste

Method

» Preheat a grill or griddle pan over medium-high heat.
» Toss the asparagus with olive oil, salt, and pepper.
» Grill for 3-4 minutes, turning occasionally, until tender and lightly charred.
» In a small pan, melt the butter and sauté the garlic for 30 seconds.
» Drizzle the garlic butter over the asparagus before serving.

Red Cabbage & Apple Sauté

Winter wonders on a plate. A slightly sweet, tangy, and crunchy side dish packed with antioxidants.

Ingredients

- » ½ red cabbage, finely shredded
- » 1 apple, julienned
- » 1 tbsp extra virgin olive oil
- » 1 tbsp apple cider vinegar
- » Sea salt & black pepper, to taste

Method

- » Heat the olive oil in a large pan over medium heat.
- » Add the cabbage and cook for 5 minutes, stirring frequently.
- » Add the apple and cook for another 2 minutes.
- » Stir in the apple cider vinegar and season with salt and pepper.
- » Serve warm or at room temperature.

Baked Sweet Potato Wedges with Smoked Paprika

An almost universal side dish. A healthier alternative to chips, packed with beta-carotene.

Ingredients

» 2 large sweet potatoes, cut into wedges
» 1 tbsp extra virgin olive oil
» 1 tsp smoked paprika
» Sea salt & black pepper, to taste

Method

» Preheat oven to 200°C (180°C fan).
» Toss the sweet potato wedges with olive oil, smoked paprika, salt, and pepper.
» Spread onto a baking tray in a single layer.
» Bake for 25-30 minutes, turning halfway, until golden and crispy on the edges.
» Serve immediately.

Sautéed Mushrooms with Thyme

A savoury, umami-rich side that pairs well with roasted meats.

Ingredients

- » 250g chestnut mushrooms, sliced
- » 1 tbsp extra virgin olive oil
- » 1 clove garlic, minced
- » 1 tsp fresh thyme leaves
- » Sea salt & black pepper, to taste

Method

- » Heat the olive oil in a frying pan over medium heat.
- » Add the mushrooms and cook for 5-6 minutes, stirring occasionally, until softened.
- » Stir in the garlic and thyme, then cook for another 2 minutes.
- » Season with salt and pepper before serving.

Now, Im not a massive fan of snacking, but if you have the right things on hand, then you can easily stay on track.

Flax & Chia Seed Crackers

I absolutely love these. Great with a cheese board too. Crispy, nutrient-dense crackers packed with omega-3s.

Ingredients

» 100g ground flaxseeds
» 50g chia seeds
» ½ tsp sea salt
» 1 tsp dried oregano
» 1 tbsp extra virgin olive oil
» 150ml water

Method

» Preheat oven to 170°C (150°C fan). Line a baking tray with parchment paper.
» In a bowl, mix flaxseeds, chia seeds, salt, and oregano. Add olive oil and water, stirring until a thick dough forms.
» Spread the dough thinly onto the lined tray using a spatula. Score into squares with a knife.
» Bake for 30-35 minutes, until crisp and golden.
» Allow to cool completely before breaking into crackers. Store in an airtight container.

Turmeric-Spiced Nuts

A crunchy, spiced snack rich in healthy fats. Need I say more.

Ingredients

» 50g walnuts
» 50g almonds
» 50g pecans
» 1 tsp turmeric

» ½ tsp ground cumin
» ½ tsp sea salt
» 1 tbsp extra virgin olive oil

Method

» Preheat oven to 180°C (160°C fan).
» In a bowl, toss the nuts with olive oil, turmeric, cumin, and salt.
» Spread onto a baking tray and roast for 10 minutes, stirring halfway through.
» Let cool before serving.

Olive Tapenade with Crudités

I adore tapenade. A savoury dip served with fresh vegetables. This is great on top of roasted salmon too.

Ingredients

» 100g black olives, pitted
» 1 clove garlic, minced
» 1 tbsp capers
» 1 tbsp extra virgin olive oil
» Juice of ½ lemon

» Sea salt & black pepper, to taste
» 1 cucumber, sliced
» 1 red pepper, sliced

Method

» Blend olives, garlic, capers, olive oil, and lemon juice into a smooth paste.
» Adjust seasoning to taste.
» Serve with cucumber and pepper slices.

Chia & Almond Butter Energy Balls

A nutritious, bite-sized snack with no added sugar.

Ingredients

- » 100g almond butter
- » 50g chia seeds
- » 50g ground flaxseeds
- » 1 tsp cinnamon
- » 1 tsp vanilla extract
- » 1 tbsp coconut oil, melted

Method

- » Mix all ingredients in a bowl until a thick dough forms.
- » Roll into small balls and refrigerate for 30 minutes until firm.
- » Store in an airtight container in the fridge.

Smoked Salmon & Cucumber Bites

A light, protein-rich snack.

Ingredients

- » 1 cucumber, sliced into rounds
- » 100g smoked salmon, cut into strips
- » 1 tbsp coconut yoghurt
- » 1 tsp fresh dill, chopped

Method

- » Top each cucumber slice with a piece of smoked salmon.
- » Add a small dollop of coconut yoghurt and sprinkle with dill.
- » Serve immediately.

Walnut & Dark Chocolate Bites

A few of these with a cup of green tea. perfect. A rich, antioxi-dant-packed treat.

Ingredients

» 50g walnuts, chopped

» 50g 85% dark chocolate, melted

Method

» Dip walnut pieces into melted dark chocolate.
» Place on parchment paper and refrigerate for 30 minutes until set.
» Store in an airtight container.

Curried Roasted Chickpeas

A crunchy, spiced snack. Who needs crisps?

Ingredients

» 1 tin chickpeas, drained and patted dry
» 1 tbsp extra virgin olive oil
» 1 tsp curry powder
» ½ tsp sea salt

Method

» Preheat oven to 200°C (180°C fan).
» Toss chickpeas with olive oil, curry powder, and salt.
» Spread onto a baking tray and roast for 25 minutes, shaking halfway.
» Let cool before serving.

Homemade Flaxseed Granola Clusters

A crunchy, omega-3-rich snack.

Ingredients

- » 100g flaxseeds
- » 50g coconut flakes
- » 1 tbsp coconut oil, melted
- » 1 tsp cinnamon

Method

- » Preheat oven to 180°C (160°C fan).
- » Mix all ingredients together.
- » Spread onto a baking tray and bake for 15 minutes, stirring half-way.
- » Let cool before breaking into clusters.

Tahini & Cinnamon Energy Bars

I do sometimes love an energy bar mid afternoon, but most are rammed with sugar. This is a big jump in the right direction. A naturally sweet and filling snack.

Ingredients

» 100g tahini
» 50g ground flaxseeds

» 1 tsp cinnamon
» 1 tsp vanilla extract

Method

» Mix all ingredients together into a thick dough.
» Press into a lined tray and refrigerate for 1 hour.
» Slice into bars and store in the fridge.

Avocado & Cacao Mousse

A creamy, sugar-free dessert alternative. With this one I recommend playing around with the amount of honey. Some avocados are more bitter than others. Taste it and see if you need more.

Ingredients

» 2 ripe avocados
» 2 tbsp cacao powder

» 2-3tsp honey
» 1 tsp vanilla extract

Method

» Blend all ingredients until smooth.
» Serve immediately or refrigerate for a firmer texture.

Turmeric-Spiced Roasted Almonds

These can get addictive.

Ingredients

» 100g almonds
» 1 tsp turmeric

» ½ tsp sea salt
» 1 tbsp extra virgin olive oil

Method

» Preheat oven to 180°C (160°C fan).
» Toss almonds with oil, turmeric, and salt.
» Roast for 10 minutes, stirring halfway.

Beetroot & Goat's Cheese Bites

Is there a better combination than beetroot, goats cheese and walnut? I mean really......is there?

Ingredients

- » 2 medium beetroots, roasted and sliced
- » 50g goat's cheese, crumbled
- » 20g walnuts, chopped

Method

- » Top beetroot slices with goat's cheese and walnuts.
- » Serve immediately.

Stuffed Dates with Almond Butter

A naturally sweet and satisfying snack. These little blighters are addictive too. One or two is enough!

Ingredients
» 8 Medjool dates, pitted

» 2 tbsp almond butter

Method
» Fill each date with a spoonful of almond butter.
» Serve immediately or chill for a firmer texture.

CHAPTER 8:

BEYOND THE DIET - HOW TO USE NUTRITIONAL SUPPLEMENTS TO ENHANCE YOUR ANTI INFLAMMATORY LIFESTYLE.

Of course, it is our diet that is the central focus of the anti-inflammatory plan outlined in this book. After all it is the food that we consume 3 times a day that will have the biggest impact upon our internal biochemistry. You have the recipes now that will get you started and introduced to the types of foods that will be the basis of your diet going forward.

But what if you want to take it up a gear? What if you want to bring even more powerful anti-inflammatory interventions into the picture? Well, this is indeed the realm of nutritional supplements. For some reason there seems to be a little resistance to supplements these days. I get that. We do see some pretty daft claims made for them. However, as a nutritionist that works clinically, they are a powerful tool that form a key part of the protocols that I develop for my clients. So, it seems only right that we bring them into play here.

What follows is a breakdown of the supplements that are the most relevant and effective when it comes to managing inflammation. For each one I will get into the science behind how they work, tell you the type and the dosage to take, and also flag any potential risks or side effects.

Let's get into it.

EPA & DHA

This one probably isn't too surprising. We've talked a lot about essential fatty acids throughout the book, and for good reason. You may have heard about people using fish oils to help with joint pain or inflammation, but we're going to take things up a notch. While fish oils work due to their EPA and DHA content, there's a big issue: the levels of these fatty acids can vary greatly between different products or even batches, which means you can't always rely on them to be consistent.

What I recommend instead is isolating the EPA and DHA themselves. These two fatty acids have powerful anti-inflammatory effects. They work mainly by changing the structure and function of cell membranes, helping to regulate the genes involved in inflammation, and influencing the production of certain lipid molecules called specialised pro-resolving mediators (SPMs) (Calder, 2017).

A key way that EPA and DHA help with inflammation is by affecting how our bodies process a specific omega-6 fatty acid called arachidonic acid (AA). This process leads to the production of substances that promote inflammation, like series 2 prostaglandins and leukotrienes, which can keep the inflammatory response going (Serhan & Chiang, 2013). EPA steps in here by competing with AA for the same enzymes, which reduces the production of those inflammatory molecules. On top of that, EPA and DHA help produce compounds like resolvins, protectins, and maresins, which actively work to calm inflammation. They do this by reducing the number of inflammatory cells that show up at the site of injury, helping clear away dead cells, and lowering the levels of inflammatory signals in the body (Basil & Levy, 2016).

EPA and DHA also work to reduce inflammation by blocking the activation of a protein called nuclear factor-kappa B (NF-κB). NF-κB is a key regulator of inflammation, controlling the expression of cytokines like TNF-α, IL-6, and IL-1β (Calder, 2017). By keeping NF-κB in check, these fatty acids help lower overall inflammation in the body, which is particularly helpful in conditions like rheumatoid arthritis, cardiovascular disease, and metabolic syndrome. DHA, in particular, plays a role in protecting the brain, keeping its cell membranes intact and potentially reducing neuroinflammation, which is linked to cognitive decline and diseases like Alzheimer's (Cutuli, 2017).

The benefits of EPA and DHA for reducing inflammation have been backed by numerous clinical trials. A large analysis by Rangel-Huerta et al. (2012) found that omega-3 supplementation significantly lowered levels of C-reactive protein (CRP), which is a key marker of inflammation in the body. Similarly, a study by Calder (2017) showed that EPA and DHA supplementation helped reduce symptoms like joint pain and stiffness in people with rheumatoid arthritis, further proving their role in reducing inflammation.

The right dose of EPA and DHA for reducing inflammation depends on a person's individual health and diet. However, general guidelines suggest a daily dose of 1,000–3,000 mg of combined EPA and DHA for inflammation management. Higher doses may be needed for chronic conditions (Calder, 2017). Some studies recommend a 2:1 ratio of EPA to DHA for optimal anti-inflammatory effects (Freund-Levi et al., 2014). However, doses above 5,000 mg per day may increase the risk of bleeding due to the mild blood-thinning effects of omega-3s.

Although EPA and DHA are generally safe, some people may experience mild digestive issues like bloating, diarrhea, or nausea, especially at higher doses (Rice et al., 2011). One of the main safety concerns with taking large amounts of omega-3s is that they can slow down blood clotting, which could be a problem for people on blood-thinning medications like warfarin or aspirin. While this effect is still debated in terms of clinical significance, it's a good idea to be cautious if you have a bleeding disorder or are preparing for surgery (Kris-Etherton et al., 2009). Omega-3s may also lower blood pressure, which can be beneficial for those with high blood pressure, but it's important to monitor the effects if you're on medication for this (Mori & Woodman, 2006).

When it comes to supplementing with EPA and DHA, the form of the oil is important for absorption. Fish oil is the most common source, but it comes in different forms: triglyceride, ethyl ester, and re-esterified triglyceride. The triglyceride and re-esterified forms are typically absorbed better than the ethyl ester form, which needs to be converted in the liver before the body can use it (Dyerberg et al., 2010). Another popular option is krill oil, which contains EPA and DHA in a form that may be easier for your body to absorb and use (Ulven & Holven, 2015). For those following a plant-based diet, algal oil is a good alternative. It's particularly rich in DHA, with some EPA content as well (Ryan et al., 2015).

One thing to be mindful of when choosing omega-3 supplements is oxidation. Omega-3s are highly susceptible to oxidation, which can create harmful compounds and reduce their effectiveness. To avoid this, look for fish oil supplements that contain antioxidants like vitamin E or astaxanthin, and make sure they're stored properly in dark, airtight containers (Kolanowski et al., 2013). It's also important to choose reputable brands that test their products for oxidation and heavy metals to ensure safety and effectiveness.

In summary, EPA and DHA are among the most well-studied and effective nutrients for managing chronic inflammation. They work by modifying how our bodies process pro-inflammatory molecules, blocking key inflammation pathways, and promoting the resolution of inflammation. Clinical evidence supports their use in managing conditions like rheumatoid arthritis, heart disease, and neuroinflammatory diseases. While they're generally safe, proper dosing is key, especially in people taking medication for blood thinning or blood pressure. Choosing a bioavailable form like triglyceride-based fish oil, krill oil, or algal oil, and ensuring the product is of high quality, will help you get the most out of these essential fatty acids.

My recommendation - 1-2 capsules per day, supplying 750mg EPA & 250mg DHA per. capsule.

DO NOT TAKE IF - you are on any anticoagulant 'blood thinner' medication. Just stick to the oily fish in the diet.

Boswelia (Frankincense)

Now here is one you may not know is a common supplement. Boswellia serrata, also known as Indian frankincense, is a powerful natural anti-inflammatory that has been studied extensively for its ability to help manage chronic inflammation. The key compounds responsible for its effects are boswellic acids, especially two specific types: 11-keto-β-boswellic acid (KBA) and 3-O-acetyl-11-keto-β-boswellic acid (AKBA). These acids are shown to strongly inhibit key inflammation pathways in the body (Ammon, 2010). One of the main ways they work is by targeting the 5-lipoxygenase (5-LOX) enzyme, which plays a central role in producing leukotrienes—chemicals that promote inflammation in conditions like rheumatoid arthritis, asthma, and inflammatory bowel disease (Siddiqui, 2011). By blocking 5-LOX, boswellic acids help reduce inflammation, offering relief from these chronic issues.

In addition to affecting the leukotriene pathway, Boswellia serrata also influences nuclear factor-kappa B (NF-κB), a protein that regulates the production of various pro-inflammatory cytokines, such as TNF-α, IL-6, and IL-1β (Roy et al., 2019). NF-κB is often overactive in chronic inflammatory diseases, including osteoarthritis, cardiovascular disease, and neuroinflammatory conditions like Alzheimer's disease. By reducing NF-κB activity, Boswellia helps lower the levels of these harmful inflammatory molecules, which can protect tissues and ease symptoms (Ammon, 2016).

The anti-inflammatory effects of Boswellia serrata have been backed by clinical studies. For instance, a trial by Kimmatkar et al. (2003) tested a Boswellia extract in patients with knee osteoarthritis and found significant improvements in pain and joint function. Similarly, a study by Gerhardt et al. (2001) showed that patients with Crohn's disease who took Boswellia extract had a notable reduction in disease activity, which was similar to the effects of conventional anti-inflammatory medications. These studies suggest that Boswellia is a useful additional treatment for managing chronic inflammation.

The recommended dosage for Boswellia serrata depends on the specific supplement and how concentrated it is in boswellic acids. Clinical trials usually recommend a dose between 300 mg to 500 mg, taken two to three times daily, with extracts that are standardised to contain 30-40% boswellic acids (Sengupta et al., 2011). Some formulations that contain higher levels of AKBA may be more effective because of its stronger anti-inflammatory properties. Also, since boswellic acids don't dissolve well in water, some products use special delivery systems, like lecithin-complexed Boswellia, to improve absorption (Kruger et al., 2008).

While Boswellia is generally safe, there are some potential side effects, though they are typically mild. These include digestive issues like nausea, acid reflux, and diarrhea (Siddiqui, 2011). Rarely, some people might experience allergic skin reactions. Long-term safety data is still limited, but Boswellia appears to be well-tolerated when taken in the recommended amounts. However, because it can affect immune responses, people with autoimmune diseases who are on immunosuppressive drugs should be cautious (Roy et al., 2019).

Boswellia can also interact with certain medications, so it's important to take care when combining it with other treatments. For instance, since Boswellia affects leukotriene production and inflammation, using it alongside non-steroidal anti-inflammatory drugs (NSAIDs) or corticosteroids could enhance its effects, but it might also increase the risk of stomach irritation (Ammon, 2010). Additionally, Boswellia has mild anticoagulant properties, meaning it could increase the effects of blood thinners like warfarin, aspirin, or clopidogrel (Sengupta et al., 2011). Anyone on these medications should consult with a healthcare provider before starting Boswellia.

When choosing a Boswellia supplement, it's important to select one that's standardised to contain at least 30-40% boswellic acids, with a focus on AKBA for its stronger action. Some supplements use special delivery systems, like phospholipid or liposomal formulations, to improve how well the body absorbs the active compounds, offering better results than traditional Boswellia extracts (Kruger et al., 2008). Proprietary formulas such as BosPure® or ApresFlex® have been developed to optimise absorption and effectiveness, making them potentially more powerful in reducing inflammation than regular Boswellia supplements.

In conclusion, Boswellia serrata is a well-researched, natural anti-inflammatory that shows great promise in treating chronic inflammation. Its unique ability to target both the 5-LOX enzyme and NF-κB pathways sets it apart from typical anti-inflammatory medications, making it an important option in integrative medicine. While it's generally safe, people taking certain medications should be mindful of possible interactions. Future studies should continue exploring its long-term safety and how it compares to pharmaceutical anti-inflammatory drugs.

My recommendation - 500mg Boswelia extract 1-2 times a day

Curcumin (turmeric extract)

We have discussed the spice and used it in the recipes. How about bringing a concentrated supplement into the programme too? Curcumin, the active compound found in the root of Curcuma longa (turmeric), has been extensively studied for its powerful anti-inflammatory effects. It works by affecting several biological pathways, with one of the key actions being the modulation of nuclear factor-kappa B (NF-κB), a protein that controls the production of various pro-inflammatory molecules. NF-κB regulates the expression of cytokines like tumour necrosis factor-alpha (TNF-α), interleukin-6 (IL-6), and interleukin-1 beta (IL-1β), which are central players in chronic inflammation (Gupta et al., 2013). By inhibiting NF-κB, curcumin helps reduce systemic inflammation, making it helpful for managing conditions like rheumatoid arthritis, inflammatory bowel disease, and metabolic syndrome (Hewlings & Kalman, 2017).

Curcumin also affects other important pathways involved in inflammation. For example, it influences the mitogen-activated protein kinase (MAPK) and Janus kinase/signal transducer and activator of transcription (JAK/STAT) pathways, both of which help regulate the inflammatory response (Kunnumakkara et al., 2017). Furthermore, curcumin boosts the activity of nuclear factor erythroid 2-related factor 2 (Nrf2), a protein that helps protect the body from oxidative stress by promoting the production of antioxidant and detoxification enzymes like heme oxygenase-1 (HO-1) and glutathione S-transferase (GST) (Scholey et al., 2021). By both reducing inflammation and supporting antioxidant defences, curcumin offers a two-pronged approach to managing chronic inflammation.

Several clinical studies support the use of curcumin to reduce inflammation. A review by Daily et al. (2016) found that curcumin supplementation significantly lowered high-sensitivity C-reactive protein (hs-CRP) levels, which is a well-known marker of inflammation. Additionally, a randomised controlled trial by Chandran and Goel (2012) found that 500 mg of curcumin three times daily was as effective as the drug diclofenac in improving pain and joint function in people with rheumatoid arthritis, suggesting that curcumin can be a natural alternative to conventional nonsteroidal anti-inflammatory drugs (NSAIDs).

The optimal dose of curcumin depends on the formulation and individual factors like metabolic rate and existing inflammation. Curcumin in its natural form has low bioavailability, meaning it isn't well absorbed by the body. This is due to its poor solubility, fast metabolism, and limited absorption in the gut (Anand et al., 2007). To address this, several enhanced formulations have been developed to improve absorption, including curcumin combined with piperine (a compound from black pepper), phospholipids, nanoparticles, and liposomes. Piperine has been shown to increase curcumin absorption by up to 2,000% by preventing its breakdown in the liver (Shoba et al., 1998). Other formulations like curcumin phytosomes (Meriva®) and nano-formulated curcumin have been shown to offer better bioavailability, making them more effective for therapeutic use (DiSilvestro et al., 2012).

Curcumin is generally considered safe and well-tolerated, but some people may experience mild side effects, such as nausea, diarrhea, and bloating, especially at higher doses (Lao et al., 2006). While rare, there are also concerns about possible liver toxicity with excessive doses, though the evidence isn't conclusive (Hewlings & Kalman, 2017). Curcumin can also affect bile secretion, so individuals with gallbladder issues should be cautious when taking it, as it may worsen symptoms of bile duct obstruction (Goel et al., 2008).

Curcumin can interact with certain medications, so it's important to consult a healthcare provider before starting supplementation. It has mild anticoagulant effects, which may increase the risk of bleeding if combined with blood-thinning drugs like warfarin, aspirin, or clopidogrel (DiSilvestro et al., 2012). Additionally, curcumin can affect the activity of cytochrome P450 enzymes, which are involved in the metabolism of several medications, including statins, antidepressants, and chemotherapy drugs (Wang et al., 2018). Therefore, individuals on these medications should be careful and speak to their doctor before adding curcumin to their routine.

When choosing a curcumin supplement, it's essential to select one that is standardised to contain at least 95% curcuminoids for maximum potency. Supplements that include bioenhanced formulations, such as those combining curcumin with piperine (BioPerine®), phospholipids (Meriva®), or micellar curcumin (NovaSOL®), offer better absorption and more consistent therapeutic effects compared to regular curcumin (Schiborr et al., 2014). These enhanced formulations are particularly beneficial for people looking to manage inflammation, as they ensure that curcumin reaches therapeutic levels in the body with lower doses.

In conclusion, curcumin is an effective natural compound for managing inflammation. It works through several pathways, including inhibiting NF-κB, modulating the MAPK and JAK/STAT pathways, and activating antioxidant defences. Clinical evidence supports its use for conditions like arthritis, metabolic syndrome, and inflammatory bowel disease. While curcumin is generally safe, it's important to use the right dose and choose formulations that enhance absorption. People taking certain medications, particularly blood thinners or those that affect liver enzymes, should be cautious and consult their healthcare provider before starting curcumin supplementation. Ongoing research will continue to explore its long-term effectiveness and potential interactions with other anti-inflammatory compounds.

My recommendation - 1000mg of curcumin daily.

DO NOT TAKE IF - you are on any anticoagulant 'blood thinner' medication.

Devils Claw

This is one that you may want to consider if you cannot get hold of curcumin. Devil's claw (Harpagophytum procumbens) is a medicinal plant native to southern Africa, known for its strong anti-inflammatory and pain-relieving properties. The key compounds responsible for its effects are harpagosides, a type of iridoid glycoside. These compounds have been studied for their ability to reduce inflammation through various mechanisms. One of the main ways devil's claw works is by inhibiting nuclear factor-kappa B (NF-κB), a protein that controls the production of pro-inflammatory cytokines like TNF-α, IL-6, and IL-1β (Fiebich et al., 2012). By reducing the activity of NF-κB, devil's claw lowers the production of these inflammatory molecules, helping to alleviate pain and inflammation in conditions like osteoarthritis, rheumatoid arthritis, and lower back pain (Chrubasik et al., 2006).

Along with NF-κB inhibition, harpagosides in devil's claw also affect the cyclooxygenase (COX) and lipoxygenase (LOX) pathways. These pathways are involved in the production of prostaglandins and leukotrienes, which are key players in inflammation (Loew & Kaszkin, 2002). Devil's claw has been shown to inhibit the COX-2 enzyme, which reduces prostaglandin production and helps ease inflammatory pain (Fiebich et al., 2001). This action is similar to how nonsteroidal anti-inflammatory drugs (NSAIDs) work, making devil's claw a good natural alternative for those who want to avoid the gastrointestinal side effects that often come with NSAIDs (Brien et al., 2006).

Clinical studies support the effectiveness of devil's claw in treating chronic inflammatory conditions. For example, a study by Chrubasik et al. (2003) found that people with osteoarthritis of the hip and knee who took devil's claw extract daily experienced less pain and better mobility. Another review by Gagnier et al. (2004) found that devil's claw was just as effective as traditional painkillers in reducing lower back pain. These results show that devil's claw can be a helpful treatment for chronic pain and inflammation, improving quality of life for those suffering from these conditions.

The recommended dosage of devil's claw depends on the extract's concentration and the severity of the condition. Clinical studies suggest that doses between 600 mg and 2,610 mg per day of a standardised extract with 50–100 mg of harpagosides are effective in reducing pain from inflammation (Mills & Bone, 2013). For more severe symptoms, higher doses may be needed, but long-term use should be monitored for safety and effectiveness. Devil's claw is commonly taken in capsules, tablets, or liquid extracts, with standardised products being preferred for consistent dosing and bioactivity.

While devil's claw is generally well-tolerated, it can cause mild side effects, especially related to digestion, like diarrhea, nausea, and stomach discomfort (Hegner et al., 2017). These effects usually go away with continued use or a change in dose. However, people with digestive issues such as peptic ulcers or GERD should be cautious, as devil's claw can increase stomach acid production, potentially worsening their symptoms (Loew & Kaszkin, 2002).

Devil's claw can also interact with some medications, so it's important to use it carefully if you're taking other drugs. Because it has mild anticoagulant effects, it can enhance the action of blood thinners like warfarin, aspirin, and clopidogrel, which could increase the risk of bleeding (Mills & Bone, 2013). People on these medications should consult their doctor before using devil's claw. Devil's claw may also affect blood sugar levels by improving insulin sensitivity, which could make diabetes medications like metformin and sulfonylureas more effective (Hegner et al., 2017). People with diabetes should monitor their blood sugar closely while using devil's claw. Additionally, devil's claw has been shown to lower blood pressure, so it may interact with antihypertensive medications, requiring careful monitoring in people taking blood pressure-lowering drugs (Brien et al., 2006).

When selecting a devil's claw supplement, it's important to choose one that is standardised to contain a known amount of harpagosides. Products with extracts containing 1.5–2% harpagosides are ideal for therapeutic use (Chrubasik et al., 2006). Liquid extracts and tinctures can also be used, but you may need to take larger doses to get the same amount of active compounds as you would from capsules or tablets. Freeze-dried or concentrated extracts are generally the best at preserving the bioactive compounds, ensuring consistent effectiveness. Choosing supplements that have been tested for purity and potency by third-party labs is also a good idea to ensure quality and reliability.

In conclusion, devil's claw is a well-researched, natural anti-inflammatory that can help with conditions like osteoarthritis, rheumatoid arthritis, and lower back pain. It works through multiple pathways, including NF-κB inhibition, COX-2 modulation, and LOX pathway suppression. Clinical evidence shows that devil's claw is as effective as conventional NSAIDs in reducing pain and inflammation, without the common side effects of NSAID use. While generally safe, it's important to be mindful of potential interactions with anticoagulants, diabetes medications, and blood pressure drugs. Choosing a standardised supplement with a verified harpagoside content ensures you get the full benefits of devil's claw. Further research will continue to explore its long-term safety and effectiveness in managing chronic inflammatory conditions.

My recommendation - 500mg extract 2 x daily

DO NOT TAKE IF - you are on any anticoagulant 'blood thinner' medication.

Vitamin D

This is one of the most commonly used supplements in the World and possibly one you are already using to some degree. Vitamin D is a fat-soluble hormone-like compound that plays an essential role in regulating immune function and inflammation. Its active form, called calcitriol (1,25-dihydroxyvitamin D3), has strong anti-inflammatory effects. It works by interacting with the vitamin D receptor (VDR), which is found in many immune cells, including macrophages, dendritic cells, and T cells (Martens et al., 2020). One of the key ways vitamin D reduces inflammation is by inhibiting the activation of nuclear factor-kappa B (NF-κB), a protein that controls the production of pro-inflammatory molecules like TNF-α, IL-6, and IL-1β (Liu et al., 2018). By suppressing NF-κB, vitamin D helps lower the production of these inflammatory markers, reducing systemic inflammation and protecting against chronic inflammatory conditions.

Along with controlling NF-κB, vitamin D also supports the function of regulatory T cells (Tregs), which are crucial for maintaining immune balance and preventing overactive immune responses (Jeffery et al., 2019). When Tregs are more active, they help reduce the inflammation caused by certain immune cells like Th1 and Th17 cells. These cells are involved in autoimmune diseases and chronic inflammatory conditions such as rheumatoid arthritis, multiple sclerosis, and inflammatory bowel disease. Vitamin D also boosts the production of anti-inflammatory molecules, including IL-10, which helps maintain immune balance and further reduce inflammation (Aranow, 2011).

Low levels of vitamin D have been linked to a higher risk of chronic inflammatory diseases. Studies show that people with low vitamin D levels are more likely to develop conditions like cardiovascular disease, metabolic syndrome, and autoimmune diseases (Holick, 2017). Supplementing with vitamin D can reduce markers of inflammation, such as C-reactive protein (CRP) and IL-6, in people who are deficient or have insufficient vitamin D (Calton et al., 2020). Clinical trials also suggest that vitamin D supplementation can reduce disease activity and improve symptoms in patients with rheumatoid arthritis, showing its potential as a supportive treatment for inflammatory diseases (Zittermann et al., 2016).

The optimal dose of vitamin D for reducing inflammation depends on factors like baseline vitamin D levels, age, body weight, and genetic differences in how the body processes vitamin D. The Endocrine Society recommends a daily intake of 1,500-2,000 IU for adults to maintain adequate vitamin D levels above 30 ng/mL (Holick et al., 2011). However, people with severe vitamin D deficiency may need higher doses, usually between 4,000-10,000 IU per day, but this should be done under medical supervision. Some research suggests that keeping vitamin D levels between 40-60 ng/mL may offer the most significant anti-inflammatory benefits (Carlberg & Haq, 2022). It's important to regularly check vitamin D levels to avoid taking too much, as excessive vitamin D can lead to toxicity.

While vitamin D is generally safe, taking too much can lead to hypercalcemia, a condition where calcium levels in the blood become too high. This can cause symptoms like nausea, vomiting, kidney stones, and calcification of soft tissues (Bouillon, 2017). The tolerable upper intake level (UL) for vitamin D set by the Institute of Medicine is 4,000 IU per day for adults, although some studies suggest that doses up to 10,000 IU per day are safe for most people without causing hypercalcemia (Vieth, 2007). People with conditions that increase the risk of hypercalcemia, such as primary hyperparathyroidism or certain granulomatous diseases like sarcoidosis, should be especially cautious, as their bodies might produce too much calcitriol, leading to high calcium levels (Adams & Hewison, 2010).

Vitamin D can interact with some medications, affecting their effectiveness or increasing the risk of side effects. Corticosteroids, commonly used for inflammation, can interfere with vitamin D metabolism, leading to deficiency and worsening inflammation (Rosen et al., 2012). Certain anticonvulsant medications, like phenytoin and carbamazepine, can also speed up the breakdown of vitamin D, raising the risk of deficiency (Holick, 2017). On the other hand, vitamin D supplementation may increase calcium absorption, which can interfere with osteoporosis treatments like bisphosphonates. People on blood-thinning medications, such as warfarin, should be mindful of their vitamin D intake, as changes in calcium metabolism could affect blood clotting (Schwalfenberg, 2015).

When it comes to supplements, vitamin D3 (cholecalciferol) is the preferred form, as it is more effective at raising vitamin D levels than D2 (ergocalciferol) (Trang et al., 1998). Vitamin D3 is better absorbed and has a longer half-life, making it a better choice for maintaining adequate levels. People with malabsorption disorders like coeliac disease or Crohn's disease may benefit from liposomal or emulsified vitamin D formulations, which improve absorption (Heaney et al., 2011). Vitamin D is also best taken with a meal that contains fat, since it is a fat-soluble vitamin (Dawson-Hughes et al., 2015).

Emerging research is exploring how vitamin D works together with other nutrients, particularly vitamin K2. Vitamin K2 helps direct calcium to bones and away from soft tissues, potentially preventing the buildup of calcium in blood vessels when taking high doses of vitamin D (Theuwissen et al., 2012). Some experts recommend that people who take high doses of vitamin D should also consider supplementing with vitamin K2 to maintain healthy calcium levels and support cardiovascular health.

Overall, vitamin D is a powerful modulator of inflammation with a well-established role in immune regulation and the prevention of chronic diseases. Its effects on NF-κB suppression, cytokine modulation, and Treg activation make it a valuable tool for managing inflammation. While vitamin D is generally safe, it's essential to use the correct dose and monitor levels to avoid toxicity. Choosing vitamin D3 over D2 and considering vitamin K2 for calcium balance may provide added benefits. Future research should continue refining optimal dosing strategies and explore the long-term effects of vitamin D supplementation in managing chronic inflammatory diseases.

My recommendation - 4000 - 8000iu daily.

Magnesium

Magnesium is an essential mineral that plays a key role in controlling inflammation and supporting immune function. It's involved in over 300 enzymatic reactions in the body, many of which help regulate inflammation, oxidative stress, and cell signaling (Costello et al., 2016). One of the main ways magnesium helps reduce inflammation is by regulating a protein called nuclear factor-kappa B (NF-κB), which controls the production of inflammatory molecules like TNF-α, IL-6, and IL-1β (Castiglioni et al., 2013). When magnesium levels are low, NF-κB becomes more active, increasing inflammation in the body. This connection has been linked to chronic health conditions such as cardiovascular disease, type 2 diabetes, and neurodegenerative disorders (Rosanoff et al., 2016).

Magnesium also affects inflammation through its influence on the NLRP3 inflammasome, a protein complex that plays a central role in the body's immune response (Weglicki, 2012). If the NLRP3 inflammasome is overactive, it can contribute to conditions like rheumatoid arthritis, inflammatory bowel disease, and metabolic syndrome. Magnesium helps by blocking the activation of this inflammasome, reducing the release of pro-inflammatory cytokines and decreasing the damage caused by chronic inflammation (Zhang et al., 2017). Additionally, magnesium acts as a calcium antagonist, meaning it helps prevent excessive calcium buildup inside cells, which can worsen inflammation and oxidative stress (Dominguez et al., 2013). By keeping calcium levels balanced, magnesium helps reduce cellular inflammation, improving immune regulation and lowering the risk of chronic diseases.

Clinical research shows that magnesium supplementation can significantly lower markers of inflammation. A meta-analysis by Dibaba et al. (2017) found that taking magnesium reduced C-reactive protein (CRP), a well-known marker of inflammation. This effect was especially noticeable in people with low magnesium levels or those dealing with chronic conditions characterized by high inflammation. Another study by Zarezadeh et al. (2020) found that magnesium supplementation improved inflammation and oxidative stress in people with metabolic syndrome, further supporting its role as an anti-inflammatory agent.

The ideal dose of magnesium for reducing inflammation depends on individual needs, diet, and magnesium levels. General guidelines suggest 300-400 mg of magnesium per day for adults, but therapeutic doses for inflammation may range from 400-800 mg per day, especially for those with magnesium deficiency or specific health conditions (Volpe, 2013). Higher doses should be used carefully, as too much magnesium, especially from supplements, can cause digestive issues like diarrhea. To avoid this, it's best to use forms of magnesium that are well absorbed, like magnesium glycinate, magnesium malate, and magnesium taurate, which tend to cause fewer digestive problems (Coudray, 2011).

While magnesium is generally safe, taking too much can lead to hypermagnesemia, a condition where magnesium levels in the blood become too high. Symptoms can include low blood pressure, nausea, tiredness, muscle weakness, and in severe cases, irregular heart rhythms (Guerrera et al., 2009). People with kidney problems, particularly those with chronic kidney disease (CKD), need to be careful with magnesium supplements because their kidneys may not be able to clear magnesium from the body as effectively (de Baaij et al., 2015). It's important for people with CKD to check with a healthcare provider before taking magnesium supplements to avoid the risk of toxicity.

Magnesium can also interact with certain medications, so it's important to take care when supplementing. Proton pump inhibitors (PPIs), which are used to treat acid reflux and gastric ulcers, can reduce magnesium absorption over time, leading to deficiency and worsening inflammation (Hess et al., 2017). People on long-term PPI therapy may need magnesium supplements to make up for this loss. Magnesium can also interfere with the absorption of some antibiotics, like tetracyclines and fluoroquinolones, by forming insoluble complexes in the gut, reducing their effectiveness (Schwalfenberg & Genuis, 2017). To avoid this, magnesium supplements should be taken at least two hours before or after antibiotics. Additionally, magnesium can enhance the effects of blood pressure-lowering drugs and calcium channel blockers, which may cause blood pressure to drop too much. People taking these medications should monitor their blood pressure while using magnesium supplements (Rosanoff et al., 2016).

The form of magnesium you take can affect how well it works. Magnesium glycinate is often recommended for its high bio-availability and gentle effect on the digestive system, making it a good choice for people who have digestive issues (Coudray, 2011). Magnesium malate is particularly helpful for people with chronic fatigue syndrome or fibromyalgia because it supports energy production in cells and muscle function (Yamamura et al., 2019). Magnesium taurate, which combines magnesium with taurine, may have extra benefits for heart health by supporting blood vessel function and reducing oxidative stress (Rosanoff et al., 2016). On the other hand, magnesium oxide, while common and inexpensive, is poorly absorbed and can cause more digestive discomfort, making it less ideal for long-term use (Coudray, 2011).

Overall, magnesium is a key nutrient for reducing inflammation and supporting immune function. Its ability to regulate NF-κB, control the NLRP3 inflammasome, and maintain calcium balance is crucial for reducing chronic inflammation and preventing related diseases. While magnesium supplementation is generally safe and effective, it's important to use the right dose and form to get the most benefit while avoiding any side effects. People with chronic inflammatory conditions, especially those at risk of magnesium deficiency, can significantly benefit from magnesium supplementation as part of a comprehensive anti-inflammatory approach.

My recommendation - 500mg magnesium glycinate 2-3 x daily. Take one of the doses an hour before bed for a deeper sleep.

Quercetin

Quercetin is a natural flavonoid found in a wide range of plant foods, including onions, apples, berries, citrus fruits, and green tea. It's been extensively studied for its anti-inflammatory effects, mainly because it can influence key pathways involved in inflammation and oxidative stress (Li et al., 2016). One of the main ways quercetin works is by inhibiting nuclear factor-kappa B (NF-κB), a protein that regulates the production of several pro-inflammatory cytokines, such as TNF-α, IL-6, and IL-1β (Zhang et al., 2019). By reducing NF-κB activity, quercetin lowers the levels of these cytokines, helping to reduce systemic inflammation and prevent the tissue damage seen in chronic inflammatory diseases.

In addition to its effect on NF-κB, quercetin also influences other pathways involved in inflammation. For example, it can inhibit the activation of mitogen-activated protein kinases (MAPKs), which are important for cellular responses to stress and inflammation (Boots et al., 2008). Specifically, quercetin blocks the activation of p38 MAPK and c-Jun N-terminal kinase (JNK), both of which are involved in diseases like rheumatoid arthritis and inflammatory bowel disease (Li et al., 2016). Furthermore, quercetin helps activate the Nrf2 pathway, which boosts the body's antioxidant defences by increasing the production of detoxifying enzymes like heme oxygenase-1 (HO-1) and glutathione S-transferase (GST) (Sinha et al., 2014). This ability to both reduce inflammation and increase antioxidant protection makes quercetin a powerful tool for managing chronic inflammatory conditions.

Clinical studies have shown that quercetin supplementation can significantly lower markers of inflammation. For example, a study by Javadi et al. (2019) found that taking 500 mg of quercetin per day for eight weeks reduced levels of high-sensitivity C-reactive protein (hs-CRP) and IL-6 in people with metabolic syndrome. Similarly, another study by Lee et al. (2016) showed that quercetin supplementation improved symptoms and reduced inflammation in individuals with rheumatoid arthritis. These results suggest that quercetin can effectively reduce inflammation in conditions where cytokine activity and oxidative stress are elevated.

The optimal dose of quercetin for reducing inflammation depends on factors like individual health status, diet, and how well the body absorbs it. While dietary sources provide small amounts, therapeutic effects typically require supplementation of 500-1,000 mg per day (Egert et al., 2012). However, quercetin is not very well absorbed on its own because it has poor water solubility and is quickly broken down in the liver and intestines (Manach et al., 2005). To improve absorption, quercetin is often combined with phospholipids, liposomes, or other bioenhancers like bromelain or vitamin C, which increase its stability and availability in the body (Nair et al., 2020). Forms like quercetin dihydrate and quercetin phytosome are some of the most bioavailable, making them ideal for therapeutic use.

Although quercetin is generally safe, high doses can cause mild digestive issues, including nausea, bloating, and diarrhea (Harwood et al., 2007). Some studies also suggest that large amounts of quercetin may interfere with thyroid function by inhibiting thyroid peroxidase, which is essential for thyroid hormone production (Shoskes et al., 2010). As a result, people with thyroid problems should be cautious when taking high doses of quercetin. Additionally, at very high doses, quercetin can act as a pro-oxidant, potentially causing oxidative stress instead of relieving it (Boots et al., 2008). To avoid this, it's best to stick to the recommended dosage and eat a diet rich in other antioxidants.

Quercetin can interact with several medications, so it's important to consider this when supplementing. It inhibits cytochrome P450 enzymes, especially CYP3A4, which can affect how the body processes various drugs, including statins, calcium channel blockers, and immunosuppressants (Gee et al., 2018). This may alter the effectiveness of these medications or increase the risk of side effects. Quercetin also has mild anticoagulant effects, meaning it can enhance the blood-thinning action of medications like warfarin and aspirin, raising the risk of bleeding (Wang et al., 2015). Anyone on blood thinners should talk to their doctor before starting quercetin supplements. Additionally, quercetin can interact with certain antibiotics, such as fluoroquinolones, by competing for absorption in the intestines, which could reduce their effectiveness (Murota & Terao, 2003). This highlights the importance of checking for potential drug-supplement interactions when using quercetin.

The form of quercetin you take can significantly affect its effectiveness. Quercetin dihydrate is one of the most stable and bioavailable forms, making it an excellent choice for supplementation (Manach et al., 2005). Quercetin phytosome, which combines quercetin with phospholipids, has been shown to improve absorption and increase its bioavailability (Nair et al., 2020). Liposomal quercetin is another advanced formulation designed to increase solubility and extend its time in the bloodstream, offering even greater therapeutic benefits (Harwood et al., 2007). To further enhance absorption, quercetin can be combined with bromelain or vitamin C.

In conclusion, quercetin is a highly effective natural compound for managing chronic inflammation. Its ability to inhibit NF-κB and MAPK pathways, along with its antioxidant properties, makes it a valuable option for conditions involving chronic inflammation. Clinical trials have shown that quercetin can reduce inflammatory markers, and its low toxicity profile makes it suitable for long-term use. However, it's important to choose a well-absorbed form, such as quercetin phytosome or liposomal quercetin, to maximize its effects. Monitoring for potential drug interactions is also crucial to ensure safe and effective use. Future research should continue to investigate the long-term effects of quercetin supplementation and its potential role in preventing and managing inflammatory diseases.

Probiotics

Probiotics are live microorganisms that provide health benefits when taken in the right amounts. They've gained a lot of attention for their ability to reduce inflammation and support immune function. Most of their anti-inflammatory effects happen through interactions with the gut microbiota, the gut lining, and the immune system. One of the main ways probiotics work is by strengthening the gut barrier, which prevents harmful substances like bacterial endotoxins (e.g., lipopolysaccharides or LPS) from entering the bloodstream. When LPS enters the circulation, it can contribute to a condition called metabolic endotoxaemia, which is linked to chronic inflammation and diseases like metabolic syndrome, cardiovascular disease, and autoimmune disorders (Cani et al., 2008). By boosting proteins that form tight junctions between gut cells, such as occludin and zonula occludens-1 (ZO-1), probiotics improve gut permeability and reduce systemic inflammation (Dai et al., 2012).

Beyond protecting the gut barrier, probiotics also help regulate immune responses by interacting with pattern recognition receptors like toll-like receptors (TLRs) and nucleotide-binding oligomerisation domain (NOD) receptors on immune and gut cells. These interactions influence the production of cytokines, shifting the immune response from a pro-inflammatory one (driven by Th1/Th17 cells) to a more anti-inflammatory one mediated by regulatory T cells (Tregs) (Ouwehand et al., 2002). Some probiotic strains, like Lactobacillus rhamnosus GG and Bifidobacterium longum, are particularly effective at increasing the production of IL-10 (an anti-inflammatory cytokine) while lowering levels of pro-inflammatory cytokines like TNF-α and IL-6 (Forsythe et al., 2007).

Certain probiotic strains also reduce inflammation by increasing the production of short-chain fatty acids (SCFAs), such as butyrate, propionate, and acetate. These SCFAs not only provide energy to the cells lining the colon but also help regulate immune function by activating G-protein coupled receptors like GPR43 and inhibiting enzymes called histone deacetylases (HDACs), which reduces inflammation (Morrison & Preston, 2016). Strains like Bifidobacterium breve and Faecalibacterium prausnitzii are particularly good at producing SCFAs and have been linked to lower levels of intestinal and systemic inflammation in conditions like inflammatory bowel disease (IBD) and irritable bowel syndrome (IBS) (Riviere et al., 2016).

Clinical studies have shown that probiotics can be effective in managing chronic inflammation. For example, a meta-analysis by Zhang et al. (2016) found that probiotic supplementation significantly reduced CRP levels, a key marker of inflammation, in people with metabolic disorders. A study by Kato-Kataoka et al. (2016) showed that Lactobacillus casei Shirota helped reduce stress-induced inflammation and improved gut barrier function in healthy people. In patients with rheumatoid arthritis, a study by Vaghef-Mehrabany et al. (2014) found that taking a multi-strain probiotic with Lactobacillus acidophilus, Lactobacillus casei, and Bifidobacterium bifidum led to big reductions in inflammatory markers and disease activity scores.

The right dose of probiotics can vary depending on the strain, health status, and the specific inflammatory condition being treated. Generally, effective doses range from 1 billion to 50 billion colony-forming units (CFU) per day, with higher doses needed for conditions like IBD and metabolic syndrome (West et al., 2017). Multi-strain formulations tend to be more effective than single-strain probiotics because they can target different parts of the gut and have a wider range of benefits. For example, Lactobacillus plantarum 299v and Bifidobacterium lactis HN019 are particularly helpful for reducing systemic inflammation and improving gut health in people with metabolic disorders (Riedel et al., 2014).

Probiotics are generally safe, but some people should be careful when using them. Those with severe immune conditions, such as people undergoing chemotherapy or organ transplants, may be at risk of infections like bacteraemia or fungaemia when taking certain probiotics, especially Saccharomyces boulardii (Ohishi et al., 2010). People with small intestinal bacterial overgrowth (SIBO) or histamine intolerance may also experience bloating and other digestive issues, especially when using strains that produce histamine, like Lactobacillus reuteri (Engelbrektson et al., 2002). In these cases, it may be better to use low-histamine strains like Bifidobacterium infantis or Lactobacillus gasseri.

Probiotics can interact with certain medications as well. They are often used alongside antibiotics to prevent antibiotic-associated diarrhea, but they should be taken at least two hours apart from antibiotics to avoid inactivating them (Goldenberg et al., 2017). Probiotics may also interact with immunosuppressive drugs like methotrexate and corticosteroids, potentially requiring dosage adjustments in people with autoimmune conditions (Liu et al., 2018). Additionally, some probiotic strains can affect serotonin metabolism, which may influence the effects of antidepressants like selective serotonin reuptake inhibitors (SSRIs) in people with depression and anxiety (Clapp et al., 2017).

When choosing a probiotic supplement, it's important to consider the strain, potency, and delivery method. Enteric-coated capsules and microencapsulated formulas are great choices because they protect the probiotics from stomach acid and bile, ensuring they reach the gut where they can have the most impact (Gueimonde et al., 2006). Fermented foods like kefir, kimchi, and sauerkraut also provide probiotics, but their bacterial content can vary greatly depending on how they're prepared. Synbiotic supplements, which combine probiotics with prebiotics (like inulin or fructo-oligosaccharides), can improve the probiotics' effectiveness by providing food for the beneficial bacteria (Kolida et al., 2002). These may be especially helpful for people with an imbalance in their gut bacteria, known as dysbiosis.

Overall, probiotics are a promising approach for managing chronic inflammation through mechanisms like improving gut barrier function, modulating immune responses, and producing anti-inflammatory SCFAs. Strains like Lactobacillus rhamnosus GG, Bifidobacterium longum, and Faecalibacterium prausnitzii have been shown to have strong anti-inflammatory effects in conditions like metabolic syndrome, IBD, and rheumatoid arthritis. While generally safe, it's important to choose a high-quality probiotic, monitor for potential interactions with medications, and adjust dosages as needed. Continued research will help clarify the long-term effects of probiotics and their role in preventing and managing inflammatory diseases.

BRINGING IT ALL TOGETHER: YOUR 6 STEP PLAN SIMPLIFIED

Before we draw to a close, I want to tie everything together that we have discussed so that you have everything in a simple couple of pages to look back to when you need reminders or just pointers of what you need to do every day. Even though we have covered a great deal and there is indeed a great deal of science behind all of this and behind all of the recommendations I have made, the execution is pretty simple. Putting it into practice is very easy when you know how. So, before I go, let's summarise the anti-inflammatory diet and how you can banish chronic inflammation for life.

Swap the white for the brown

One of the most powerful swaps that you can make in your every day diet, is centred around the types of carbohydrates that you choose. By simply swapping your everyday carbohydrate staples like bread and rice for the brown versions, you get multiple relevant benefits.

Firstly, because of their higher fibre content and the time they take to digest, they release their glucose content far more slowly. This keeps blood glucose levels even and prevents blood sugar spikes and the associated insulin spikes. Not only does high blood glucose and insulin affect our energy levels, mental clarity and cause us to put on weight. It is also fuel for the inflammatory flame. It drives and aggravates chronic inflammation.

I should also remind you that it is really worth while cutting down your overall starchy carb intake by about half. Use the perfect plate diagram to guide you. Eating this way will really keep blood sugar under control, and opens up even more space for more beneficial ingredients.

Also opt for other carbohydrate sources such as sweet potatoes, squash, and legumes. These are very low glycemic, high in fibre and packed with a whole host of beneficial phytochemicals.

The final benefit of this simple swap is that these high fibre carbohydrate sources are an amazing food source for our microbiome. They feed on them, reproduce in number, and also secrete beneficial by products that improve the health of the gut. Remember, if the gut health starts to slide, it can impact systemic inflammation and upset many key immunological responses. Feeding the microbiome with high fibre foods will strengthen it and improve every aspect of gut health overall.

Get Fat Smart

The next step is a vital one. We need to get fat smart, and cut out the fats that seem to dominate our modern diets that are directly fuelling inflammation. Our modern diet of processed foods and the supposed 'heart healthy' vegetable oils are just an inflammatory time bomb - and the explosions have begun.

Your focus here is to cut out rich sources of the omega 6 fatty acids, and trans fats. Omega 6 fatty acids are vital in very small amounts that are easy to get. Any more than the small amount that we need and we will start to manufacture more of the pro inflammatory eicosanoids such as series 2 prostaglandins. By cutting them out, and incorporating the next step, we minimise the production of pro inflammatory eicosanoids and increase the production of the anti-inflammatory eicosanoids.

So what are you cutting out? Avoid the following:

- » *Omega 6 Dominant Oils:*
- » Soybean oil
- » Corn oil
- » Sunflower oil
- » Safflower oil
- » Cottonseed oil
- » Grapeseed oil
- » Peanut oil
- » Sesame oil
- » Rice bran oil
- » Canola oil
- » Walnut oil
- » *And trans fats such as:*
- » Partially hydrogenated oil
- » Hydrogenated vegetable oil
- » Vegetable shortening
- » Margarine (unless specified as trans-fat-free)
- » Hydrogenated palm oil
- » Hydrogenated soybean oil
- » Hydrogenated cottonseed oil
- » Hydrogenated rapeseed oil
- » Hydrogenated sunflower oil
- » Hydrogenated corn oil
- » Mono- and diglycerides (can contain trans fats, though not always)
- » Interesterified fats

The easiest way to do all of this is to cook from scratch as often as is feasibly possible. When you do, do not use an omega 6 rich oil. Use extra virgin olive oil (that is mostly omega 9 which has no influence on inflammation) or coconut oil sparingly. Simple!

Up the three

The next step on from what I have just discussed is to increase your intake of omega 3. Especially the long chain omega 3 fatty acids EPA & DHA from oily fish and the right supplements. These will feed directly into the metabolic pathways that manufacture the anti-inflammatory eicosanoids such as series 1 and series 3 prostaglandins, and other substances such as resolvins. These actively turn inflammation off. If we are consuming less of the oils that are turned into pro inflammatory compounds and more of the oils that are turned into the anti inflammatory compounds, then we force the body's hand. We tilt things in our favour.

Whilst plant sources of omega 3 such as ALA are very poorly converted into EPA and DHA, they do assist with reducing inflammation, because they occupy the same enzymes that omega 6 fatty acids use for their conversion. The more omega

3 fatty acids that occupy these enzymes, the less omega 6 will get a look in. So, they assist the process, even if it is less potently. This is why you have seen some plant sources of omega 3 such as flax and walnuts in the recipes section. It all helps.

How do we achieve all of this? Eat more oily fish such as salmon, mackerel, herrings and sardines. Add flax, chia, walnuts etc to your diet, and of course take targeted supplements to really amplify things.

Get fresh. Get Whole. get Colourful

Now, as our focus is absolutely cooking from scratch, this is a perfect chance to make use of as many brightly coloured fruit and veg as possible. Remember, the vibrant colours are made by phytochemicals that are anti oxidant and anti-inflammatory. Load up on these as much as you can.

The simple rule here - make half of your plate at each meal, brightly coloured non starchy vegetables. Load them up to fill your body with an abundance of these powerful anti-inflammatory

Spice up your plate

The next step on from what I have just discussed is to increase your intake of anti-inflammatory spices. Certain spices contain powerful bioactive compounds that directly influence inflammatory pathways, helping to dampen excessive inflammation and support overall metabolic balance. Curcumin, the active compound in turmeric, for example, has been shown to inhibit the activity of pro-inflammatory enzymes such as COX-2 and LOX, much like some pharmaceutical anti-inflammatories, but without the side effects. Other compounds, such as the gingerols in ginger, have similar effects, actively reducing the production of inflammatory cytokines and supporting the resolution of inflammation.

If we are consuming fewer inflammatory triggers from processed foods and more of the compounds that block inflammatory pathways, we shift the body's response in our favour. We actively create an internal environment that is less prone to chronic inflammation. Even smaller amounts consumed regularly can make a meaningful impact over time. This is why you will see spices such as turmeric, ginger, cinnamon, and cloves appearing throughout the recipes in this book—they all contribute to the bigger picture.

How do we achieve all of this? Use more turmeric in cooking, ideally combined with black pepper to enhance absorption. Add fresh or dried ginger to meals, teas, or smoothies. Make liberal use of cinnamon and cloves in both savoury and sweet dishes. And, of course, if needed, targeted supplements can help provide an extra anti-inflammatory boost.

Supplement Smart

Then the final step in all of this is to use targeted supplements to really amplify things further. While diet lays the foundation, the right supplements can provide a concentrated dose of the key compounds that drive down inflammation and support the body's natural healing processes. For example, high-quality EPA & DHA supplements ensure a reliable intake of these crucial long-chain omega-3s, feeding directly into the pathways that generate anti-inflammatory mediators like resolvins and protectins. Curcumin, in a well-absorbed form such as a liposomal or phytosomal supplement, can work far more effectively than dietary turmeric alone, actively blocking inflammatory enzymes and cytokines.

Quercetin, a powerful flavonoid found in foods like onions and apples, stabilises immune cells and helps to regulate histamine, making it a great tool for inflammation linked to allergies and immune overactivity. Magnesium plays a critical role too, helping to modulate stress responses, relax blood vessels, and lower inflammation at a cellular level. Then there's

Vitamin D—arguably one of the most essential anti-inflammatory nutrients of all. Low levels are linked to a whole host of inflammatory conditions, and supplementing can be an absolute game-changer, especially in those who are deficient. And let's not forget probiotics. A well-balanced microbiome plays a huge role in immune regulation, gut integrity, and overall inflammatory balance, making the right strains of beneficial bacteria a key part of the puzzle.

How do we achieve all of this? First, focus on food—always. But then, where needed, bring in supplements that are well-formulated and clinically relevant. A good omega-3 supplement, a bioavailable curcumin, a high-quality magnesium, vitamin D3 at appropriate levels, and a well-chosen probiotic can all take things to the next level. It's about stacking the odds in your favour, giving your body the best possible support to fight inflammation effectively.

Additional Lifestyle Factors for Long-Term Anti-Inflammatory Living

While diet and supplements are fundamental, anti-inflammatory living extends beyond what's on your plate or in your supplement routine. The following lifestyle practices are essential for keeping inflammation in check over the long term.

1. Regular Exercise

Exercise is one of the most effective ways to reduce chronic inflammation. Regular physical activity, such as walking, swimming, or cycling, helps reduce inflammation by promoting the release of anti-inflammatory molecules and improving immune function. Aim for at least 30 minutes of moderate exercise most days of the week. Not only does this reduce inflammation, but it also supports cardiovascular health, improves insulin sensitivity, and enhances mood.

2. Stress Management

Chronic stress is a significant contributor to inflammation. The body's stress response involves the release of cortisol, a hormone that, when elevated over prolonged periods, can exacerbate inflammation. Incorporating stress-reduction practices such as meditation, yoga, deep breathing, and mindfulness into your daily routine can help reduce the production of stress hormones and lower inflammation.

3. Quality Sleep

Adequate, restful sleep is essential for maintaining a healthy immune system and reducing inflammation. Poor sleep has been shown to increase levels of inflammatory cytokines in the body. Aim for 7-9 hours of quality sleep each night, and create a restful sleep environment by keeping your bedroom cool, dark, and free of distractions like screens.

4. Healthy Body Weight

Excess body fat, particularly visceral fat (fat around the organs), is a major contributor to chronic inflammation. Maintaining a healthy weight through a balanced diet and regular exercise is essential for keeping inflammation at bay. Even small reductions in body fat can have a significant impact on reducing inflammation and improving overall health.

5. Hydration

Drinking enough water is crucial for keeping your body's inflammatory processes in check. Dehydration can stress the body, contributing to inflammation. Aim to drink at least 8 glasses of water per day, and adjust your intake based on your activity level and climate.

Sustaining Anti-Inflammatory Living Over Time

One of the most important aspects of this approach is sustainability. A truly anti-inflammatory lifestyle isn't about strict rules or perfection, but about making choices that you can sustain for the rest of your life. Think of it as creating a routine that you enjoy and that feels aligned with your long-term health goals. It's about balancing indulgence with discipline, recognising when your body needs extra nourishment, and knowing when to take a break from routine.

This is the key to creating lifelong habits that support anti-inflammatory health. The flexibility to make adjustments, based on your unique needs and circumstances, will ensure that the process feels natural and not overwhelming.

Remember, the goal isn't to "fix" yourself—it's to create lasting, healthy habits that support your body's natural ability to manage inflammation. When you do this, you're investing in a future where inflammation is no longer a silent threat to your health but something you can control and minimise over time.

Looking Ahead: A Future Free from Chronic Inflammation

As we conclude this book, I want to leave you with a sense of empowerment and possibility. The battle against chronic inflammation isn't a fight you're facing alone. The tools, knowledge, and strategies you've gained throughout this journey are now in your hands, and they're ready to guide you toward a healthier, more vibrant life. With the right mindset and the commitment to make small changes each day, you can create a future that is free from the limitations of chronic disease.

By adopting an anti-inflammatory lifestyle, you're not just improving your own health—you're helping to shift the tide of modern disease prevention. Every choice you make ripples outward, helping to create a world where health is prioritized, inflammation is managed, and disease is no longer inevitable.

As you move forward, remember that you are in control of your health. You have the power to shape your future through the decisions you make today. Make those decisions wisely, with love and respect for your body, and watch as you build a life full of vitality, free from the grip of chronic inflammation.

CONCLUSION

So there we are. You have all of the tools now at your disposal to drive down chronic inflammation and take proactive steps towards safe guarding your future health. That is what I really want from this. I want you to understand that you can absolutely be proactive in your healthcare. This is not a passive journey. You don't just have to be in the hands of the gods. You can take steps every single day to fight back. The food that we choose to eat will influence our internal biochemistry. It will affect every conceivable chemical reaction, and tissue, and body system. Whether it affects these positively or negatively entirely depends upon what passes our lips. The key is to understand what are the good choices to make and what ones are relevant for us.

Your health does not just happen to you. You are not exclusively your genetics or the victim of circumstance. You can take action.

So, get out there and make a change. Put this information into practice and watch the change happen. Watch the wisdom of your body jump into action.

REFERENCES

Chapter 2: The Impact Of Chronic Inflammation On Health

- Barnes, P.J. (2008). Immunology of asthma and chronic obstructive pulmonary disease. *Nature Reviews Immunology*, 8(3), pp.183-192.

- Capuron, L. & Miller, A.H. (2011). Immune system to brain signaling: neuropsychopharmacological implications. *Pharmacology & Therapeutics*, 130(2), pp.226-238.

- Colotta, F., Allavena, P., Sica, A., Garlanda, C., & Mantovani, A. (2009). Cancer-related inflammation, the seventh hallmark of cancer: links to genetic instability. *Carcinogenesis*, 30(7), pp.1073-1081.

- Dowlati, Y., Herrmann, N., Swardfager, W., et al. (2010). A meta-analysis of cytokines in major depression. *Biological Psychiatry*, 67(5), pp.446-457.

- Epa, R., Pariante, C.M., & Mondelli, V. (2021). The role of peripheral inflammation in clinical response to psychotropic treatment in depression: a systematic review. *Frontiers in Psychiatry*, 12, p.715-734.

- Foster, J.A. & McVey Neufeld, K.A. (2013). Gut-brain axis: how the microbiome influences anxiety and depression. *Trends in Neurosciences*, 36(5), pp.305-312.

- Haapakoski, R., Mathieu, J., Ebmeier, K.P., Alenius, H., & Kivimäki, M. (2015). Cumulative meta-analysis of interleukins 6 and 1β, tumour necrosis factor α and C-reactive protein in patients with major depressive disorder. *Brain, Behavior, and Immunity*, 49, pp.206-215.

- Heneka, M.T., Golenbock, D.T., & Latz, E. (2015). Innate immunity in Alzheimer's disease. *Nature Immunology*, 16(3), pp.229-236.

- Hirsch, E.C., & Hunot, S. (2009). Neuroinflammation in Parkinson's disease: a target for neuroprotection? *The Lancet Neurology*, 8(4), pp.382-397.

- Holmes, S.E., Hinz, R., Conen, S., et al. (2018). Elevated translocator protein density is associated with chronic low-grade inflammation in depression. *Neuropsychopharmacology*, 43(7), pp.1552-1559.

- Hotamisligil, G.S. (2006). Inflammation and metabolic disorders. *Nature*, 444(7121), pp.860-867.

- Köhler, O., Benros, M.E., Nordentoft, M., et al. (2014). Effect of anti-inflammatory treatment on depression, depressive symptoms, and adverse effects: a systematic review and meta-analysis of randomized clinical trials. *JAMA Psychiatry*, 71(12), pp.1381-1391.

- Libby, P. (2012). Inflammation in atherosclerosis. *Arteriosclerosis, Thrombosis, and Vascular Biology*, 32(9), pp.2045-2051.

- Miller, A.H. & Raison, C.L. (2016). The role of inflammation in depression: from evolutionary imperative to modern treatment target. *Nature Reviews Immunology*, 16(1), pp.22-34.

- Raison, C.L., Capuron, L., & Miller, A.H. (2006). Cytokines sing the blues: inflammation and the pathogenesis of depression. *Trends in Immunology*, 27(1), pp.24-31.

- Setiawan, E., Wilson, A.A., Mizrahi, R., et al. (2015). Role of translocator protein density, a marker of neuroinflammation, in the brain during major depressive episodes. *JAMA Psychiatry*, 72(3), pp.268-275.

- Smolen, J.S., Aletaha, D., & McInnes, I.B. (2016). Rheumatoid arthritis. *The Lancet*, 388(10055), pp.2023-2038.

- Ungaro, R., Mehandru, S., Allen, P.B., Peyrin-Biroulet, L., & Colombel, J.F. (2017). Ulcerative colitis. *The Lancet*, 389(10080), pp.1756-1770.

- Weisberg, S.P., et al. (2003). Obesity is associated with macrophage accumulation in adipose tissue. *Journal of Clinical Investigation*, 112(12), pp.1796-1808.

- Wium-Andersen, M.K., Ørsted, D.D., Nielsen, S.F., & Nordestgaard, B.G. (2013). Elevated C-reactive protein levels, psychological distress, and depression in 73,131 individuals. *JAMA Psychiatry*, 70(2), pp.176-184.

- Ye, J. (2013). Mechanisms of insulin resistance in obesity. *Frontiers in Medicine*, 7(1), pp.14-24.

Chapter 3: The Non Dietary Lifestyle Drivers Of Chronic Inflammation

- Adler, N.E. & Newman, K. (2002). Socioeconomic disparities in health: pathways and policies. *Health Affairs*, 21(2), pp.60-76.

- Agus, A., Planchais, J., & Sokol, H. (2018). Gut microbiota regulation of tryptophan metabolism in health and disease. *Cell Host & Microbe*, 23(6), 716-724.

- Barnes, P.J. (2008). The cytokine network in chronic obstructive pulmonary disease. *American Journal of Respiratory Cell and Molecular Biology*, 38(3), pp.232-238.

- Beavers, K.M., Brinkley, T.E., & Nicklas, B.J. (2010). Effect of exercise training on chronic inflammation. *Clinical Geriatric Medicine*, 26(4), pp.597-611.

- Brook, R.D., Rajagopalan, S., Pope, C.A., Brook, J.R., Bhatnagar, A., & Diez-Roux, A.V. (2010). Particulate matter air pollution and cardiovascular disease: an update to the scientific statement from the American Heart Association. *Circulation*, 121(21), pp.2331-2378.

- Cani, P.D., Amar, J., Iglesias, M.A., Poggi, M., Knauf, C., Bastelica, D., ... & Burcelin, R. (2007). Metabolic endotoxemia initiates obesity and insulin resistance. *Diabetes*, 56(7), 1761-1772.

- Cedernaes, J., Schiöth, H.B., & Benedict, C. (2019). Determinants of shortened, disrupted, and mistimed sleep and associated metabolic health consequences in healthy humans. *Diabetes*, 68(5), pp.819-829.

- Coussens, L.M. & Werb, Z. (2002). Inflammation and cancer. *Nature*, 420(6917), pp.860-867.

- Cryan, J.F., & Dinan, T.G. (2012). Mind-altering microorganisms: the impact of the gut microbiota on brain and behaviour. *Nature Reviews Neuroscience*, 13(10), 701-712.

- Danese, A. & Lewis, S.J. (2017). Psychoneuroimmunology of early-life stress: the hidden wounds of childhood trauma? *Neuropsychopharmacology*, 42(1), pp.99-114.

- Fasano, A. (2011). Leaky gut and autoimmune diseases. *Clinical Reviews in Allergy & Immunology*, 42(1), 71-78.

- Fasano, A. (2012). Intestinal permeability and its regulation by zonulin: diagnostic and therapeutic implications. *Clinical Gastroenterology and Hepatology*, 10(10), 1096-1100.

- Furman, D., Campisi, J., Verdin, E., et al. (2019). Chronic inflammation in the etiology of disease across the life span. *Nature Medicine*, 25(12), pp.1822-1832.

- Furusawa, Y., Obata, Y., Fukuda, S., Endo, T.A., Nakato, G., Takahashi, D., ... & Ohno, H. (2013). Commensal microbe-derived butyrate induces the differentiation of colonic regulatory T cells. *Nature*, 504(7480), 446-450.

- Gleeson, M., Bishop, N.C., Stensel, D.J., Lindley, M.R., Mastana, S.S., & Nimmo, M.A. (2011). The anti-inflammatory effects of exercise: mechanisms and implications for the prevention and treatment of disease. *Nature Reviews Immunology*, 11(9), pp.607-615.

- Hawkley, L.C. & Cacioppo, J.T. (2003). Loneliness and pathways to disease. *Brain, Behavior, and Immunity*, 17(Suppl 1), pp.S98-S105.

- Irwin, M.R. (2015). Why sleep is important for health: a psychoneuroimmunology perspective. *Annual Review of Psychology*, 66, pp.143-172.

- Kivimäki, M. & Steptoe, A. (2018). Effects of stress on the development and progression of cardiovascular disease. *Nature Reviews Cardiology*, 15(4), pp.215-229.

- Kostic, A.D., Howitt, M.R., & Garrett, W.S. (2014). Exploring host-microbiota interactions in animal models and humans. *Genes & Development*, 27(7), 701-718.

- López, P., de Paz, B., Rodríguez-Carrio, J., Hevia, A., & Suárez, A. (2021). Impact of gut microbiota on autoimmune diseases: a complex question. *Autoimmunity Reviews*, 20(8), 102820.

- Patisaul, H.B. & Adewale, H.B. (2009). Long-term effects of environmental endocrine disruptors on reproductive physiology and behavior. *Frontiers in Behavioral Neuroscience*, 3, p.10.

- Slavich, G.M. & Irwin, M.R. (2014). From stress to inflammation and major depressive disorder: a social signal transduction theory of depression. *Psychological Bulletin*, 140(3), pp.774-815.

- Szabo, G. & Saha, B. (2015). Alcohol's effect on host defense. *Alcohol Research: Current Reviews*, 37(2), pp.159-170.

• Tchounwou, P.B., Yedjou, C.G., Patlolla, A.K., & Sutton, D.J. (2012). Heavy metal toxicity and the environment. *Molecular, Clinical and Environmental Toxicology*, 101, pp.133-164.

• Turnbaugh, P.J., Ley, R.E., Mahowald, M.A., Magrini, V., Mardis, E.R., & Gordon, J.I. (2006). An obesity-associated gut microbiome with increased capacity for energy harvest. *Nature*, 444(7122), 1027-1031.

• Weisberg, S.P., et al. (2003). Obesity is associated with macrophage accumulation in adipose tissue. *Journal of Clinical Investigation*, 112(12), pp.1796-1808.

• Yaggi, H.K., Concato, J., Kernan, W.N., Lichtman, J.H., Brass, L.M., & Mohsenin, V. (2005). Obstructive sleep apnea as a risk factor for stroke and death. *New England Journal of Medicine*, 353(19), pp.2034-2041.

Chapter 5: The Foods That Fuel The Fire

• Baer, D.J., Judd, J.T., Clevidence, B.A., et al. (2004). Dietary fatty acids affect endothelial function in healthy men. *The Journal of Nutrition*, 134(4), pp.874-879.

• Bishehsari, F., Magno, E., Swanson, G., Desai, V., & Voigt, R.M. (2017). Alcohol and gut-derived inflammation. *Alcohol Research: Current Reviews*, 38(2), pp.163-171.

• Calder, P.C. (2017). Omega-3 fatty acids and inflammatory processes: from molecules to man. *Biochemical Society Transactions*, 45(5), pp.1105-1115.

• Cani, P.D., Amar, J., Iglesias, M.A., et al. (2007). Metabolic endotoxemia initiates obesity and insulin resistance. *Diabetes*, 56(7), pp.1761-1772.

• Ceriello, A. (2005). Postprandial hyperglycemia and diabetes complications: is it time to treat? *Diabetes*, 54(1), pp.1-7.

- Crews, F.T., Sarkar, D.K., Qin, L., et al. (2017). Neuroimmune function and the consequences of alcohol exposure. *Alcohol Research: Current Reviews*, 38(2), pp.331-341.

- Esposito, K., Nappo, F., Marfella, R., et al. (2002). Inflammatory cytokine concentrations are acutely increased by hyperglycemia in humans. *Diabetes Care*, 25(3), pp.560-563.

- Fasano, A. (2012). Leaky gut and autoimmune diseases. *Clinical Reviews in Allergy & Immunology*, 42(1), pp.71-78.

- Gebauer, S.K., Psota, T.L., Kris-Etherton, P.M. & Baer, D.J. (2007). Effects of different dietary saturated fatty acids on plasma lipid and lipoprotein levels in healthy subjects. *The American Journal of Clinical Nutrition*, 86(1), pp.66-75.

- Goldin, A., Beckman, J.A., Schmidt, A.M. & Creager, M.A. (2006). Advanced glycation end products: sparking the development of diabetic vascular injury. *Circulation*, 114(6), pp.597-605.

- Hotamisligil, G.S. (2006). Inflammation and metabolic disorders. *Nature*, 444(7121), pp.860-867.

- Mozaffarian, D., Katan, M.B., Ascherio, A., Stampfer, M.J., & Willett, W.C. (2006). Trans fatty acids and cardiovascular disease. *The New England Journal of Medicine*, 354(15), pp.1601-1613.

- Rooks, M.G. & Garrett, W.S. (2016). Gut microbiota, metabolites and host immunity. *Nature Reviews Immunology*, 16(6), pp.341-352.

- Shoelson, S.E., Lee, J. & Goldfine, A.B. (2006). Inflammation and insulin resistance. *The Journal of Clinical Investigation*, 116(7), pp.1793-1801.

- Simopoulos, A.P. (2016). An increase in the omega-6/omega-3 fatty acid ratio increases the risk for obesity. *Nutrients*, 8(3), p.128.

- Softic, S., Cohen, D.E. & Kahn, C.R. (2017). Role of dietary fructose and hepatic de novo lipogenesis in fatty liver disease. *Digestive Diseases and Sciences*, 62(5), pp.1282-1293.

- Szabo, G. & Saha, B. (2015). Alcohol's effect on host defense. *Alcohol Research: Current Reviews*, 37(2), pp.159-170.

- Uribarri, J., Woodruff, S., Goodman, S., et al. (2010). Advanced glycation end products in foods and a practical guide to their reduction. *Journal of the American Dietetic Association*, 110(6), pp.911-916.

- Vlassara, H. & Striker, G.E. (2011). Advanced glycation end-products in diabetes and diabetic complications. *Endocrinology and Metabolism Clinics of North America*, 40(4), pp.875-890.

- Wang, H.J., Gao, B., & Zakhari, S. (2010). The role of gut-liver axis in alcohol-induced liver injury. *Nature Reviews Gastroenterology & Hepatology*, 7(4), pp.237-247.

- Wellen, K.E. & Hotamisligil, G.S. (2005). Inflammation, stress, and diabetes. *The Journal of Clinical Investigation*, 115(5), pp.1111-1119.

- Willett, W.C., Stampfer, M.J., Manson, J.E., et al. (1993). Intake of trans fatty acids and risk of coronary heart disease among women. *The Lancet*, 341(8845), pp.581-585.

Chapter 6: The Anti-Inflammatory Foods To Power Your Plate

- Bazan, N.G. (2018). Omega-3 fatty acids, pro-inflammatory signaling, and neuroprotection. *Molecular Neurobiology*, 55(9), pp.7063-7075.

- Brenna, J.T., et al. (2009). Alpha-linolenic acid supplementation and conversion to n-3 long-chain polyunsaturated fatty acids in humans. *Prostaglandins, Leukotrienes & Essential Fatty Acids*, 80(2-3), pp.85-91.

- Calder, P.C. (2017). Omega-3 fatty acids and inflammatory processes: from molecules to man. *Biochemical Society Transactions*, 45(5), pp.1105-1115.

- Minihane, A.M., Vinoy, S., Russell, W.R., et al. (2016). Low-grade inflammation, diet composition, and health: current research evidence and its translation. *British Journal of Nutrition*, 116(1), pp.1-14.

- Mozaffarian, D. & Wu, J.H. (2012). Omega-3 fatty acids and cardiovascular disease. *Journal of the American College of Cardiology*, 58(20), pp.2047-2067.

- Serhan, C.N. & Chiang, N. (2013). Resolution phase lipid mediators of inflammation: agonists of resolution. *Current Opinion in Pharmacology*, 13(4), pp.632-640.

- Simopoulos, A.P. (2016). An increase in the omega-6/omega-3 fatty acid ratio increases the risk for obesity. *Nutrients*, 8(3), p.128.

- Basu, A., Rhone, M. and Lyons, T.J. (2010) 'Strawberries, blueberries, and cranberries in the metabolic syndrome: Clinical perspectives', Journal of Agricultural and Food Chemistry, 58(7), pp. 3869-3875.

- Borges, G., Ottaviani, J.I., Crozier, A., and Ensunsa, J.L. (2018) 'Grapefruit polyphenols and their bioavailability: Role in inflammation and metabolism', Food & Function, 9(6), pp. 3038-3045.

- Calder, P.C. (2021) 'Diet, immunity and inflammation', BMJ Nutrition, Prevention & Health, 4(1), pp. 74-84.

- Clifford, T., Howatson, G., West, D.J. and Stevenson, E.J. (2015) 'The potential benefits of red beetroot supplementation in health and disease', Nutrients, 7(4), pp. 2801-2822.

- Ellis, C.L., Edirisinghe, I., Kappagoda, T. and Burton-Freeman, B. (2011) 'Attenuation of meal-induced inflammatory and thrombotic responses in overweight men and women after 6-week daily strawberry (Fragaria) intake', Journal of Atherosclerosis and Thrombosis, 18(4), pp. 318-327.

- Estruel-Amades, S., Camps-Bossacoma, M., Massot-Cladera, M. et al. (2019) 'Raspberry consumption improves intestinal and systemic immunity-related parameters in healthy rats', Food & Function, 10(1), pp. 452-463.

- Frémont, L. (2000) 'Biological effects of resveratrol', Life Sciences, 66(8), pp. 663-673.

- Ghanim, H., Sia, C.L., Abuaysheh, S., Green, K. et al. (2011) 'An anti-inflammatory and reactive oxygen species suppressive effects of naringenin in human subjects', Journal of Clinical Endocrinology & Metabolism, 96(9), pp. 3537-3545.

- Gill, C.I.R., Boyd, A., McDermott, E. et al. (2017) 'Potential anti-inflammatory effects of pomegranate and its constituents in colorectal cancer', European Journal of Nutrition, 56(2), pp. 417-425.

- Grosso, G., Stepaniak, U., Micek, A. et al. (2017) 'Dietary polyphenols and inflammation: Results from the Polish arm of the HAPIEE study', European Journal of Nutrition, 56(4), pp. 1409-1420.

- Guo, X., Tresserra-Rimbau, A., Estruch, R. et al. (2020) 'Effects of polyphenol consumption on cardiovascular risk factors: A randomized trial of citrus flavonoids', The American Journal of Clinical Nutrition, 111(6), pp. 1299-1307.

- Jia, H., Liu, J., Zhu, X. et al. (2020) 'Naringenin attenuates inflammation in diabetic nephropathy by modulating the TLR4/NF-κB signaling pathway', Phytomedicine, 67, 153147.

- Kim, D.O., Jeong, S.W. and Lee, C.Y. (2013) 'Antioxidant capacity of phenolic phytochemicals from various plums', Food Chemistry, 81(3), pp. 321-326.

- Lima, G.P., Vianello, F., Corrêa, C.R. et al. (2019) 'Polyphenols in fruits and vegetables and its effect on human health', Food & Nutrition Research, 63(1), 1581080.

- Li, Y., Zhang, J.J., Xu, D.P. et al. (2016) 'Bioactivities and health benefits of wild fruits', International Journal of Molecular Sciences, 17(8), pp. 1258.

- Li, Y., Fang, H., Xu, W. et al. (2018) 'The role of resveratrol in cancer therapy', International Journal of Molecular Sciences, 19(7), pp. 1918.

- Meydani, M. and Hasan, S.T. (2010) 'Dietary polyphenols and obesity', Nutrients, 2(7), pp. 737-751.

- Meydani, M., Anthoni, U., Scott, T. et al. (2012) 'Effects of blueberries on biomarkers of inflammation and endothelial dysfunction in overweight men and women: A randomized controlled trial', Journal of Nutrition, 142(2), pp. 181-186.

- Norberto, S., Silva, S., Meireles, M. et al. (2013) 'Blueberry anthocyanins in health promotion', Molecules, 18(2), pp. 1422-1456.

- Peluso, I., Miglio, C., Morabito, G. et al. (2018) 'Flavonoids and immune function', Molecular Aspects of Medicine, 61, pp. 17-24.

- Poulsen, M.M., Vestergaard, P.F., Clasen, B.F.F. et al. (2013) 'High-dose resveratrol supplementation in obese men: An investigator-initiated, randomized, placebo-controlled clinical trial of substrate metabolism, insulin sensitivity, and body composition', Diabetes, 62(4), pp. 1186-1195.

- Rao, A.V. and Agarwal, S. (1999) 'Role of antioxidant lycopene in cancer and heart disease', Journal of the American College of Nutrition, 19(5), pp. 563-569.

- Rodriguez-Mateos, A., Rendeiro, C., Bergillos-Meca, T. et al. (2013) 'Blueberry intervention improves vascular function and decreases inflammation in healthy men', Molecular Nutrition & Food Research, 57(7), pp. 1124-1131.

- Seeram, N.P. (2008) 'Berry fruits: Compositional elements, biochemical activities, and the impact of their intake on human health, performance, and disease', Journal of Agricultural and Food Chemistry, 56(3), pp. 627-629.

- Shukitt-Hale, B., Cheng, V. and Joseph, J.A. (2009) 'Effects of blackberries on motor and cognitive function in aged rats', Nutritional Neuroscience, 12(3), pp. 135-140.

- Siervo, M., Lara, J., Ogbonmwan, I. and Mathers, J.C. (2013) 'Inorganic nitrate and beetroot juice supplementation reduces blood pressure in adults: A systematic review and meta-analysis', Journal of Nutrition, 143(6), pp. 818-826.

- Sies, H. and Stahl, W. (2017) 'Nutritional protection against skin damage from sunlight', Annual Review of Nutrition, 24, pp. 173-200.

- Trombold, J.R., Barnes, J.N., Critchley, L. and Coyle, E.F. (2010) 'Ellagitannin consumption improves strength recovery 2-3 days after eccentric exercise', Medicine & Science in Sports & Exercise, 42(3), pp. 493-498.

- Van den Abbeele, P., Belzer, C., Goossens, M. et al. (2011) 'Butyrate-producing Clostridium cluster XIVa species contribute to bioavailability of anthocyanins', Nutrition & Metabolism, 8(1), pp. 5.

- Wu, H., Ha, T., Liu, L. et al. (2015) 'Red cabbage anthocyanins suppress inflammation in vitro and in vivo', Journal of Agricultural and Food Chemistry, 63(23), pp. 5103-5111.

- Burgos-Morón, E., Calderón-Montaño, J.M., Salvador, J., Robles, A. and López-Lázaro, M., 2021. The dark side of curcumin. *International Journal of Molecular Sciences*, 22(2), p.726.

- Chainani-Wu, N., 2018. Safety and anti-inflammatory activity of curcumin: a component of turmeric (*Curcuma longa*). *The Journal of Alternative and Complementary Medicine*, 19(5), pp. 435-442.

- Feng, W., Wang, H., Zhang, P., Gao, C., Tao, J., Ge, Z. and Wang, X., 2020. Modulation of gut microbiota contributes to curcumin-mediated attenuation of LPS-induced inflammation. *Food & Function*, 11(10), pp. 9358-9369.

- Gupta, S.C., Patchva, S. and Aggarwal, B.B., 2021. Therapeutic roles of curcumin: lessons learned from clinical trials. *The AAPS Journal*, 15(1), pp.195-218.

- Jurenka, J.S., 2009. Anti-inflammatory properties of curcumin, a major constituent of *Curcuma longa*: a review of preclinical and clinical research. *Alternative Medicine Review*, 14(2), pp. 141-153.

- Sharma, R.A., Steward, W.P. and Gescher, A.J., 2020. Pharmacokinetics and pharmacodynamics of curcumin. *The Molecular Targets and Therapeutic Uses of Curcumin in Health and Disease*, pp. 453-470.

- Aggarwal, B.B. & Shishodia, S. (2006) *Molecular targets and therapeutic uses of spices: Modern uses for ancient medicine*. Singapore: World Scientific.

- Bae, S.H., Yoo, H., Lee, S.R. & Lee, S. (2014) 'The antioxidant properties of hot pepper (Capsicum annuum) seed extract and its preventive effect on lipid peroxidation in muscle of microfilleted fish cake', *Journal of Food Quality*, 37, pp. 1–8.

- Bahamondes, P., Vargas, M., Riveros, C. & Sandoval, J. (2016) 'Chemical composition and antimicrobial and antioxidant activities of allspice essential oil (Pimenta dioica (L.) Merr.)', *Natural Product Communications*, 11, pp. 1133–1136.

- Basch, E., Ulbricht, C., Kuo, G., Szapary, P. & Smith, M. (2003) 'Therapeutic applications of fenugreek (Trigonella foenum-graecum L.)', *Alternative Medicine Review*, 8(1), pp. 20–27.

- Cao, H., Polansky, M.M. & Anderson, R.A. (2018) 'Cinnamon extract and polyphenols affect the expression of tristetraprolin, proinflammatory cytokines, and migration of monocytes', *Journal of Nutrition & Intermediary Metabolism*, 14, pp. 29–34.

- Chaieb, K., Hajlaoui, H., Zmantar, T., Kahla-Nakbi, A.B., Rouabhia, M., Mahdouani, K. & Bakhrouf, A. (2007) 'The chemical composition and biological activity of clove essential oil, Eugenia caryophyllata (Syzigium aromaticum L. Myrtaceae): A short review', *Phytotherapy Research*, 21(6), pp. 501–506.

- Cortés-Rojas, D.F., de Souza, C.R.F. & Oliveira, W.P. (2014) 'Clove (Syzygium aromaticum): a precious spice', *Asian Pacific Journal of Tropical Biomedicine*, 4(2), pp. 90–96.

- Elbetieha, A., Da'as, S.I., Khamas, W. & Darmani, H. (2014) 'Evaluation of the toxic potentials of Laurus nobilis (laurel) in rats', *Journal of Ethnopharmacology*, 151(3), pp. 1149–1152.

- Esposito, K., Nappo, F., Giugliano, F., Di Palo, C., Ciotola, M., Barbieri, M. et al. (2002) 'Cytokine milieu tends toward inflammation in type 2 diabetes', *Diabetes Care*, 25(2), pp. 364–368.

- Fahey, J.W., Zhang, Y. & Talalay, P. (2001) 'Broccoli sprouts: an exceptionally rich source of inducers of enzymes that protect against chemical carcinogens', *Proceedings of the National Academy of Sciences*, 94(19), pp. 10367–10372.

- Faudale, M., Viladomat, F., Bastida, J., Poli, F. & Codina, C. (2008) 'Antioxidant activity and phenolic composition of wild populations of *Foeniculum vulgare* Mill. from different habitats', *Food Chemistry*, 119(4), pp. 1292–1299.

- Gharby, S., Harhar, H., Guillaume, D., Haddad, A., Matthäus, B. & Charrouf, Z. (2014) 'Chemical and oxidative properties of cumin seed oil and its fractions', *European Journal of Lipid Science and Technology*, 116(2), pp. 160–165.

- Güllüce, M., Sökmen, M., Daferera, D., Sökmen, A., Polissiou, M., Adıgüzel, A. & Özkan, H. (2004) 'In vitro antibacterial, antifungal, and antioxidant activities of the essential oil and methanol extracts of herbal parts and callus cultures of *Satureja hortensis L.*', *Journal of Agricultural and Food Chemistry*, 51(14), pp. 3958–3965.

- Imparl-Radosevich, J., Deas, S., Polansky, M.M., Baedke, D.A., Ingebritsen, T.S., Anderson, R.A. & Graves, D.J. (1998) 'Regulation of PTP-1 and insulin receptor kinase by fractions from cinnamon: Implications for cinnamon regulation of insulin signalling', *Hormone Research*, 50(3), pp. 177–182.

- Jafari, M., Gharehbeglou, P. & Hajnorouzali Tehrani, Z. (2017) 'Cardamom: A traditional healing herb with a promising potential in modern industry', *Food & Nutrition Research*, 61(1), pp. 136-176.

- Joo, J.H. & Jung, S.J. (2014) 'Pharmacological effects of capsaicin on the inflammatory responses related to obesity', *Journal of Bioscience and Bioengineering*, 118(5), pp. 266–270.

- Kashani, L., Eslatmanesh, S., Saedi, N. et al. (2018) 'Assessment of saffron (Crocus sativus L.) in the treatment of mild to moderate depression: A pilot double-blind randomized clinical trial', *Pharmacopsychiatry*, 51(4), pp. 156–164.

- Kim, S.J., Min, H.S., Kim, J.H. & Kwon, S. (2011) 'Antioxidative and antimutagenic activities of various paprika powders', *Journal of the Korean Society of Food Science and Nutrition*, 40(1), pp. 72–76.

- Lee, R. & Balick, M.J. (2005) 'Sweet wood: Traditional uses of cinnamon in Paraguay', *Economic Botany*, 59(4), pp. 395–407.

- Lee, Y., Surh, Y. & Skin, A. (2013) 'Capsaicin in red peppers: A spice with potent thermogenic effect', *Critical Reviews in Food Science and Nutrition*, 53(6), pp. 658–675.

- Ma, H., Zhao, W., Shi, N. & Yu, H. (2015) 'Effects of Capsicum annuum L. extracts on pro-inflammatory cytokines in lipopolysaccharide-induced inflammation', *Journal of Food Biochemistry*, 39(2), pp. 139–147.

- Meghwal, M. & Goswami, T.K. (2012) 'Chemical composition, nutritional, medicinal and functional properties of black pepper: A review', *Open Access Scientific Reports*, 1(2), pp. 1–5.

- Neelakantan, N., Narayanan, M., de Souza, R.J. & van Dam, R.M. (2014) 'Effect of fenugreek (Trigonella foenum-graecum L.) intake on glycemia: A meta-analysis of clinical trials', *Nutrition Journal*, 13, pp. 7–18.

- Olajide, O.A., Ajayi, A.M. & Ekhelar, A.I. (2009) 'Anti-inflammatory properties of nutmeg (Myristica fragrans)', *Pharmaceutical Biology*, 47(7), pp. 609–613.

- Peter, K.V. & Gandhi, D. (2017) 'Spices and flavor technology', in J. Chen & M. Rosenthal (eds.) *Handbook of Food Processing: Food Preservation*. Boca Raton: CRC Press, pp. 507–516.

- Piaru, S., Mahmud, R., Majid, A., Ismail, S. & Manap, M.Y. (2012) 'Chemical composition, antioxidant and cytotoxicity activities of the essential oils of Myristica fragrans and Morinda citrifolia', *Journal of Science of Food and Agriculture*, 92(3), pp. 593–597.

- Poma, A., Fontecchio, G., Carlucci, G. & Chichiricco, G. (2012) 'Anti-inflammatory properties of drugs from saffron crocus', *Anti-Inflammatory & Anti-Allergy Agents in Medicinal Chemistry*, 11(1), pp. 37–51.

- Rasool, M. & Varalakshmi, P. (2006) 'Immunomodulatory role of eugenol in adjuvant-induced arthritis: Effect on structural modification of chondrocytes', *Molecular and Cellular Biochemistry*, 292(1-2), pp. 133–137.

- Sadeghi, Z., Kuhestani, K. & Abdollahi, M. (2014) 'Cinnamon: A systematic review of adverse events', *Clinical Medicine Insights: Arthritis and Musculoskeletal Disorders*, 7, pp. 33–40.

- Sharma, R., Mathur, M., Gupta, S. & Bharati, N. (2020) 'Phytochemical properties and traditional uses of Cumin (*Cuminum cyminum L.*)', *Journal of Pharmacognosy and Phytochemistry*, 9(3), pp. 2081–2086.

- Shan, B., Cai, Y.-Z., Sun, M. & Corke, H. (2005) 'Antioxidant capacity of 26 spice extracts and characterization of their phenolic constituents', *Journal of Agricultural and Food Chemistry*, 53(20), pp. 7749–7759.

- Shoelson, S.E., Herrero, L. & Naaz, A. (2006) 'Obesity, inflammation, and insulin resistance', *Gastroenterology*, 132(6), pp. 2169–2180.

- Shoba, G., Joy, D., Joseph, T., Majeed, M., Rajendran, R. & Srinivas, P.S. (1998) 'Influence of piperine on the pharmacokinetics of curcumin in animals and human volunteers', *Planta Medica*, 64(4), pp. 353–356.

- Srinivasan, K. (2007) 'Black pepper and its pungent principle-piperine: A review of diverse physiological effects', *Critical Reviews in Food Science and Nutrition*, 47(8), pp. 735–748.

- Sundaresan, P.R., Karthikeyan, M., Deepika, D. & Tamilselvi, K. (2013) 'Protective effect of cardamom on high fat diet induced hyperlipidemia in rats', *Journal of Acute Medicine*, 3, pp. 75–81.

- Topuz, A. & Ozdemir, F. (2007) 'Assessment of carotenoids, capsaicinoids, and ascorbic acid composition of paprika produced from chilis (Capsicum annuum L.) grown in Turkey', *Journal of Agricultural and Food Chemistry*, 55(2), pp. 7190–7196.

- Traka, M. & Mithen, R. (2009) 'Glucosinolates, isothiocyanates and human health', *Phytochemistry Reviews*, 8(1), pp. 269–282.

- Warrier, S., Dorling, J. & Varma, A. (2021) 'Effect of coriander seed extracts on TNF-alpha and IL-1beta levels in a rat model', *Journal of Inflammation Research*, 14, pp. 11–19.

- Whiting, S., Derbyshire, E., Tiwari, B. & Capsa, K. (2012) 'Capsaicinoids and weight management: A comprehensive review of the evidence', *Critical Reviews in Food Science and Nutrition*, 52(2), pp. 1–16.

- Yang, Z., Yu, X., Cheng, L. & Zhang, T. (2015) 'Anti-inflammatory and immune-regulatory effect of shikimic acid in mice', *International Immunopharmacology*, 28(1), pp. 100–106.

- Zare, R., Ghiasvand, R., Feizi, A., Shokri, A. & Bahreini, M. (2019) 'Cinnamon may have therapeutic benefits on lipid profile, liver enzymes, insulin resistance, and high-sensitivity C-reactive protein levels in nonalcoholic fatty liver disease patients', *Nutrition Research*, 63, pp. 99–106.

- Ackermann, R.T., Mulrow, C.D., Ramirez, G., Gardner, C.D., Morbidoni, L. and Lawrence, V.A. (2001) 'Garlic shows promise for lowering total cholesterol', *Annals of Internal Medicine*, 135(4), pp. 277–293.

- Aggarwal, B.B. and Shishodia, S. (2006) *Molecular targets and therapeutic uses of spices: Modern uses for ancient medicine*. Singapore: World Scientific.

- Ali, B.H., Blunden, G., Tanira, M.O. and Nemmar, A. (2008) 'Some phytochemical, pharmacological and toxicological properties of ginger (Zingiber officinale Roscoe): A review of recent research', *Food and Chemical Toxicology*, 46(2), pp. 409–420.

- Altman, R.D. and Marcussen, K.C. (2001) 'Effects of a ginger extract on knee pain in patients with osteoarthritis', *Arthritis & Rheumatism*, 44(11), pp. 2531–2538.

- Amagase, H., Petesch, B.L., Matsuura, H., Kasuga, S. and Itakura, Y. (2001) 'Intake of garlic and its bioactive components', *The Journal of Nutrition*, 131(3), pp. 955S–962S.

- Asdaq, S.M.B., Fattepur, S., Dhamanigi, S.S. and Malsure, P. (2022) 'Garlic: A review of its nutritional properties, stability, and metabolic effects', *Critical Reviews in Food Science and Nutrition*, 62(4), pp. 844–854.

- Banerjee, S.K., Mukherjee, P.K. and Maulik, S.K. (2003) 'Garlic as an antioxidant: The good, the bad and the ugly', *Phytotherapy Research*, 17(2), pp. 97–106.

- Bayan, L., Koulivand, P.H. and Gorji, A. (2014) 'Garlic: A review of potential therapeutic effects', *Avicenna Journal of Phytomedicine*, 4(1), pp. 1–14.

- Black, C.D. and O'Connor, P.J. (2010) 'Acute effects of dietary ginger on muscle pain induced by eccentric exercise', *The Journal of Pain*, 11(9), pp. 894–903.

- Dhawan, V. and Jain, S. (2005) 'Effect of garlic supplementation on oxidized low density lipoproteins and lipid peroxidation in patients of essential hypertension', *Molecular and Cellular Biochemistry*, 275(1-2), pp. 85–94.

- El-Batayneh, K.M., Alnusair, M.M., El-Metwally, H.A. and Megahed, H.A. (2020) 'Potential anti-inflammatory and antioxidant activity of garlic in adjuvant arthritic rats', *Veterinary World*, 13(5), pp. 941–947.

- Grzanna, R., Lindmark, L. and Frondoza, C.G. (2005) 'Ginger—an herbal medicinal product with broad anti-inflammatory actions', *Journal of Medicinal Food*, 8(2), pp. 125–132.

- Gupta, S.C., Patchva, S., Koh, W. and Aggarwal, B.B. (2013) 'Discovery of curcumin, a component of golden spice, and its miraculous biological activities', *Clinical and Experimental Pharmacology & Physiology*, 39(3), pp. 283–299.

- Hewlings, S.J. and Kalman, D.S. (2017) 'Curcumin: A review of its effects on human health', *Foods*, 6(10), pp. 92–105.

- Kunnumakkara, A.B., Bordoloi, D., Padmavathi, G., Monisha, J., Roy, N.K., Prasad, S. and Aggarwal, B.B. (2016) 'Curcumin, the golden nutraceutical: multitargeting for multiple chronic diseases', *British Journal of Pharmacology*, 174(11), pp. 1325–1348.

- Mahluji, S., Attari, V.E., Mobasseri, M., Payahoo, L., Khajebishak, Y. and Ostadrahimi, A. (2013) 'Effects of ginger (Zingiber officinale) on plasma glucose level, HbA1c, and insulin sensitivity in type 2 diabetic patients', *International Journal of Food Sciences and Nutrition*, 64(6), pp. 682–686.

- Menon, V.P. and Sudheer, A.R. (2007) 'Antioxidant and anti-inflammatory properties of curcumin', in Aggarwal, B.B., Surh, Y.J. and Shishodia, S. (eds.) *The molecular targets and therapeutic uses of curcumin in health and disease*. New York: Springer, pp. 105–125.

- Na, L.X., Li, Y., Pan, H.Z., Zhou, X.L., Sun, D.J., Meng, M., Li, X.X. and Sun, C.H. (2011) 'Curcumin improves insulin resistance in skeletal muscle of rats', *Nutrition, Metabolism and Cardiovascular Diseases*, 21(7), pp. 526–533.

- Ng, Q.X., Koh, S.S.H., Chan, H.W. and Ho, C.Y.X. (2020) 'Clinical use of curcumin in gingivitis: A mini systematic review', *BMC Complementary Medicine and Therapies*, 20, pp. 1–7.

- Rahmani, A.H., Alzohairy, M.A., Aly, S.M. and Khan, M.A. (2014) 'Curcumin: A potential candidate in prevention of cancer via modulation of molecular pathways', *BioMed Research International*, 2014, pp. 1–15.

- Rivlin, R.S. (2001) 'Historical perspective on the use of garlic', *The Journal of Nutrition*, 131(3), pp. 951S–954S.

- Sharma, R.A., Gescher, A.J. and Steward, W.P. (2005) 'Curcumin: The story so far', *European Journal of Cancer*, 41(13), pp. 1955–1968.

- Shoba, G., Joy, D., Joseph, T., Majeed, M., Rajendran, R. and Srinivas, P.S. (1998) 'Influence of piperine on the pharmacokinetics of curcumin in animals and human volunteers', *Planta Medica*, 64(4), pp. 353–356.

- Sobenin, I.A., Myasoedova, V.A., Orekhov, A.N. (2010) 'Pharmacotherapy of atherosclerosis: seeking for clinical consensus', *International Journal of Preventive Medicine*, 1(4), pp. 256–266.

- Aggarwal, B.B. and Shishodia, S. (2006) *Molecular targets and therapeutic uses of spices: Modern uses for ancient medicine*. Singapore: World Scientific.

- Aviram, M. and Dornfeld, L. (2001) 'Pomegranate juice consumption inhibits serum angiotensin converting enzyme activity and reduces systolic blood pressure', *Atherosclerosis*, 158(1), pp. 195–198.

- Bailey, D.G., Dresser, G. and Arnold, J.M. (2013) 'Grapefruit–medication interactions: Forbidden fruit or avoidable consequences?', *CMAJ*, 185(4), pp. 309–316.

- Basu, A., Du, M., Leyva, M.J., Sanchez, K., Betts, N.M., Wu, M. and Lyons, T.J. (2010) 'Blueberries decrease cardiovascular risk factors in obese men and women with metabolic syndrome', *Journal of Nutrition*, 140(9), pp. 1582–1587.

- Bell, P.G., McHugh, M.P., Stevenson, E. and Howatson, G. (2014) 'The role of cherries in exercise and health', *Scandinavian Journal of Medicine & Science in Sports*, 24(3), pp. 477–490.

- Bischoff, S.C. (2011) 'Gut health: A new objective in medicine?', *BMC Medicine*, 9, p. 24.

- Black, P.H. and Garbutt, L.D. (2002) 'Stress, inflammation and cardiovascular disease', *Journal of Psychosomatic Research*, 52(1), pp. 1–23.

- Baur, J.A. and Sinclair, D.A. (2006) 'Therapeutic potential of resveratrol: The in vivo evidence', *Nature Reviews Drug Discovery*, 5(6), pp. 493–506.

- Burkhardt, S., Tan, D.X., Manchester, L.C., Hardeland, R. and Reiter, R.J. (2001) 'Detection and quantification of the antioxidant melatonin in Montmorency and Balaton tart cherries (Prunus cerasus)', *Journal of Agricultural and Food Chemistry*, 49(10), pp. 4898–4902.

- Carr, A.C. and Maggini, S. (2017) 'Vitamin C and immune function', *Nutrients*, 9(11), p. 1211.

- Clifford, T., Howatson, G., West, D.J. and Stevenson, E.J. (2015) 'The potential benefits of red beetroot supplementation in health and disease', *Nutrients*, 7(4), pp. 2801–2822.

- Esposito, K., Nappo, F., Giugliano, F., Di Palo, C., Ciotola, M., Barbieri, M. and Giugliano, D. (2002) 'Cytokine milieu tends toward inflammation in type 2 diabetes', *Diabetes Care*, 25(2), pp. 364–368.

- Estruel-Amades, S., Massot-Cladera, M., Pérez-Cano, F.J., Franch, À., Castell, M. and Camps-Bossacoma, M. (2019) 'Hesperidin effects on gut microbiota and gut-associated lymphoid tissue in healthy mice', *Nutrients*, 11(2), p. 324.

- Franklin, M., Bu, S.Y., Lerner, M.R., Lancaster, E.A., Bellmer, D., Brackett, D.J., Turner, N.D. and Arjmandi, B.H. (2006)

'Dried plum prevents bone loss in a male osteoporosis model via IGF-I and the RANK pathway', *Bone*, 39(6), pp. 1331–1342.

- Gerster, H. (1997) 'The potential role of lycopene for human health', *Journal of the American College of Nutrition*, 16(2), pp. 109–126.

- Giampieri, F., Tulipani, S., Alvarez-Suarez, J.M., Quiles, J.L., Mezzetti, B. and Battino, M. (2012) 'The strawberry: Composition, nutritional quality, and impact on human health', *Nutrition*, 28(1), pp. 9–19.

- Gil, M.I., Tomás-Barberán, F.A., Hess-Pierce, B. and Kader, A.A. (2000) 'Antioxidant capacities, phenolic compounds, carotenoids, and vitamin C contents of nectarine, peach, and plum cultivars from California', *Journal of Agricultural and Food Chemistry*, 50(17), pp. 4976–4982.

- Häkkinen, S.H. and Törrönen, A.R. (2000) 'Content of flavonols and selected phenolic acids in strawberries and Vaccinium species: Influence of cultivar, cultivation site and technique', *Food Research International*, 33(6), pp. 517–524.

- Hannum, S.M. (2004) 'Potential impact of strawberries on human health: A review of the science', *Critical Reviews in Food Science and Nutrition*, 44(1), pp. 1–17.

- He, J. and Giusti, M.M. (2010) 'Anthocyanins: Natural colorants with health-promoting properties', in De La Rosa, L.A., Alvarez-Parrilla, E. and González-Aguilar, G.A. (eds.) *Fruit and vegetable phytochemicals: Chemistry, nutritional value, and stability*. Chichester: Wiley-Blackwell, pp. 641–673.

- Hobbs, D.A., Goulding, M.G., Nguyen, A., Malaver, T., Walker, C.F. and Givens, D.I. (2012) 'Acute ingestion of beetroot bread increases endothelium-independent vasodilation and lowers blood pressure in healthy men: A randomized controlled trial', *The Journal of Nutrition*, 143(9), pp. 1399–1405.

- Hyson, D.A. (2011) 'A comprehensive review of apples and apple components and their relationship to human health', *Advances in Nutrition*, 2(5), pp. 408–420.

- Kalt, W., Liu, Y., McDonald, J.E., Vinqvist-Tymchuk, M.R., Fillmore, S.A.E., Zhang, Y. and Milbury, P.E. (2020) 'Anthocyanin content and profile within and among blueberry species', *Canadian Journal of Plant Science*, 100(4), pp. 374–386.

- Kelly, G.S. (2011) 'Quercetin. Monograph', *Alternative Medicine Review*, 16(2), pp. 172–194.

- Lachman, J., Orsák, M. and Pivec, V. (2020) 'Antioxidants and fruit color in red onion cultivars grown in Czech Republic', *Scientia Horticulturae*, 15(1), pp. 227–236.

- Lundberg, J.O., Weitzberg, E., Cole, J.A. and Benjamin, N. (2008) 'Nitrate, bacteria and human health', *Nature Reviews Microbiology*, 2(7), pp. 593–602.

- Middleton, E., Kandaswami, C. and Theoharides, T.C. (2000) 'The effects of plant flavonoids on mammalian cells: Implications for inflammation, heart disease, and cancer', *Pharmacological Reviews*, 52(4), pp. 673–751.

- Mohanraj, R. and Sivasankar, S. (2014) 'Sweet potato (Ipomoea batatas [L.] Lam) a valuable medicinal food: A review', *Journal of Medicinal Food*, 17(7), pp. 733–741.

- Nakatani, N., Kayano, S., Kikuzaki, H., Sumimoto, K. and Katagiri, K. (2000) 'Mitigation of oxidative damage in LDL by chlorogenic acid or plums (Prunus salicina Lindl.)', *Journal of Agricultural and Food Chemistry*, 48(11), pp. 5512–5515.

- Nile, S.H. and Park, S.W. (2014) 'Edible berries: Bioactive components and their effect on human health', *Nutrition*, 30(2), pp. 134–144.

- Rodriguez-Mateos, A., Rendeiro, C., Bergillos-Meca, T., Tabatabaee, S., George, T.W., Heiss, C. and Spencer, J.P. (2013) 'Intake and time dependence of blueberry flavonoid–induced improvements in vascular function: A randomized, controlled, double-blind, crossover intervention study with mechanistic insights into biological activity', *American Journal of Clinical Nutrition*, 98(5), pp. 1179–1191.

- Rozenberg, O., Howell, A., Aviram, M. (2006) 'Pomegranate juice sugar fraction reduces macrophage oxidative stress, and atherogenic modifications: The protective role of the unique pomegranate phenolics', *Journal of Agricultural and Food Chemistry*, 54(8), pp. 2344–2350.

- Schmidt, T., Schlemmer, B., Struckmann, C., Kirschbaum, C. and Heberle-Bors, E. (2014) 'Influence of dried plums on intestinal microflora', *Gut Microbes*, 1(2), pp. 117–123.

- Seelinger, G., Merfort, I. and Schempp, C.M. (2008) 'Anti-oxidant, anti-inflammatory and anti-allergic activities of luteolin', *Planta Medica*, 74(14), pp. 1667–1677.

- Shi, J. and Le Maguer, M. (2000) 'Lycopene in tomatoes: Chemical and physical properties affected by food processing', *Critical Reviews in Food Science and Nutrition*, 40(1), pp. 1–42.

- Tanumihardjo, S.A. (2013) 'Vitamin A and bone health: The balancing act', *Journal of Clinical Densitometry*, 16(4), pp. 414–419.

- Teow, C.C., Truong, V.D., McFeeters, R.F., Thompson, R.L., Pecota, K.V. and Yencho, G.C. (2007) 'Antioxidant activities, phenolic and β-carotene contents of sweet potato genotypes with varying flesh colours', *Food Chemistry*, 103(3), pp. 829–838.

- Traka, M. and Mithen, R. (2009) 'Glucosinolates, isothiocyanates and human health', *Phytochemistry Reviews*, 8(1), pp. 269–282.

- U.S. Department of Agriculture (2020) 'Dietary Guidelines for Americans 2020–2025', *U.S. Department of Health and Human Services*. Available at: https://www.dietaryguidelines.gov/ (Accessed: 15 February 2025).

- Wu, X., Beecher, G.R., Holden, J.M., Haytowitz, D.B., Gebhardt, S.E. and Prior, R.L. (2004) 'Lipophilic and hydrophilic antioxidant capacities of common foods in the United States', *Journal of Agricultural and Food Chemistry*, 52(12), pp. 4026–4037.

- Zafra-Stone, S., Yasmin, T., Bagchi, M., Chatterjee, A., Vinson, J.A. and Bagchi, D. (2007) 'Berry anthocyanins as novel antioxidants in human health and disease prevention', *Molecular Nutrition & Food Research*, 51(6), pp. 675–683.

Chapter 8 - Beyond The Diet - How To Use Nutritional Supplements To Enhance Your Anti Inflammatory Lifestyle.

- Ammon, H.P., 2010. Modulation of the immune system by Boswellia serrata extracts and boswellic acids. *Phytomedicine*, 17(11), pp.862-867.

- Ammon, H.P., 2016. Boswellic acids and their role in chronic inflammatory diseases. *Advances in Experimental Medicine and Biology*, 928, pp.291-327.

- Gerhardt, H., Seifert, F., Buvari, P., Vogelsang, H. and Repges, R., 2001. Therapy of active Crohn disease with Boswellia serrata extract H 15. *Zeitschrift für Gastroenterologie*, 39(01), pp.11-17.

- Kimmatkar, N., Thawani, V., Hingorani, L. and Khiyani, R., 2003. Efficacy and tolerability of Boswellia serrata extract in treatment of osteoarthritis of knee–a randomized double-blind placebo-controlled trial. *Phytomedicine*, 10(1), pp.3-7.

- Kruger, P., Vickers, A., Wiesemann, F. and Gerhards, J., 2008. Influence of phospholipid-based formulation of Boswellia extract on bioavailability and inflammation. *European Journal of Clinical Pharmacology*, 64(5), pp.455-462.

- Roy, S., Khanna, S., Krishnaraju, A.V., Hayashi, T., Bagchi, D., Bagchi, M. and Sen, C.K., 2019. Regulation of inflammatory pathways by Boswellia and curcumin: A synergistic approach to chronic inflammatory diseases. *Molecular Nutrition & Food Research*, 63(9), p.1801297.

- Sengupta, K., Alluri, K.V., Satish, A.R., Mishra, S., Golakoti, T., Sarma, K.V. and Dey, D., 2011. A double blind, randomized, placebo controlled study of the efficacy and safety of 5-Loxin for improvement of joint function in osteoarthritis. *Arthritis Research & Therapy*, 10(4), p.R85.

- Siddiqui, M.Z., 2011. Boswellia serrata, a potential anti-inflammatory agent: an overview. *Indian Journal of Pharmaceutical Sciences*, 73(3), pp.255-261.

- Adams, J.S. and Hewison, M., 2010. Update in vitamin D. *Journal of Clinical Endocrinology & Metabolism*, 95(2), pp.471-478.

- Aranow, C., 2011. Vitamin D and the immune system. *Journal of Investigative Medicine*, 59(6), pp.881-886.

- Bouillon, R., 2017. Comparative analysis of nutritional guidelines for vitamin D. *Nature Reviews Endocrinology*, 13(8), pp.466-479.

- Calton, E.K., Keane, K.N., Newsholme, P. and Soares, M.J., 2020. The impact of vitamin D levels on inflammatory status: A systematic review of immune cell studies. *PLOS ONE*, 15(1), p.e0227562.

- Carlberg, C. and Haq, A., 2022. The concept of the personal vitamin D response index. *Frontiers in Endocrinology*, 13, p.827342.

- Dawson-Hughes, B., Harris, S.S., Lichtenstein, A.H., Dolni-kowski, G., Palermo, N.J. and Rasmussen, H., 2015. Dietary fat increases vitamin D3 absorption. *Journal of the Academy of Nutrition and Dietetics*, 115(2), pp.225-230.

- Holick, M.F., 2017. Vitamin D deficiency. *New England Journal of Medicine*, 357(3), pp.266-281.

- Martens, P.J., Gysemans, C. and Verstuyf, A., 2020. Vitamin D's effect on immune function. *Nutrients*, 12(5), p.1248.

- Castiglioni, S., Cazzaniga, A., Albisetti, W. and Maier, J.A., 2013. Magnesium and osteoporosis: current state of knowledge and future research directions. *Nutrients*, 5(8), pp.3022-3033.

- Costello, R.B., Nielsen, F. and Coughlin, J., 2016. Magnesium and health outcomes: an evidence-based review. *Advances in Nutrition*, 7(2), pp.368-370.

- Coudray, C., 2011. The role of magnesium in human health and disease. *Frontiers in Bioscience*, 3(2), pp.928-939.

- Dibaba, D.T., Xun, P., Song, Y. and He, K., 2017. The effect of magnesium supplementation on C-reactive protein levels: A systematic review and meta-analysis of randomized controlled trials. *European Journal of Clinical Nutrition*, 71(8), pp.1024-1032.

- Dominguez, L.J., Veronese, N., Barbagallo, M., 2013. Magnesium and hypertension in old age. *Nutrients*, 5(10), pp.3952-3971.

- Guerrera, M.P., Volpe, S.L. and Mao, J.J., 2009. Therapeutic uses of magnesium. *American Family Physician*, 80(2), pp.157-162.

- Hess, M.W., Hoenderop, J.G. and Bindels, R.J., 2017. Systemic and renal handling of magnesium. *Clinical Kidney Journal*, 10(1), pp.52-64.

- Rosanoff, A., Weaver, C.M. and Rude, R.K., 2016. Magnesium and anti-inflammatory activity: an update. *Magnesium Research*, 29(1), pp.1-10.

- Zhang, W., Sun, W. and Wang, S., 2017. Magnesium supplementation improves inflammation in metabolic syndrome. *Journal of Translational Medicine*, 15(1), p.15.

- Boots, A.W., Haenen, G.R. and Bast, A., 2008. Health effects of quercetin: from antioxidant to nutraceutical. *European Journal of Pharmacology*, 585(2-3), pp.325-337.

- Egert, S., Bosy-Westphal, A., Seiberl, J., Kürbitz, C., Settler, U., Plachta-Danielzik, S., Wagner, A.E., Frank, J., Schrezenmeir, J. and Rimbach, G., 2012. Quercetin reduces systolic blood pressure and plasma oxidised low-density lipoprotein concentrations in overweight subjects. *Journal of Nutrition*, 139(6), pp.1022-1028.

- Javadi, F., Khademi, F., Godazandeh, G., Alipour, F. and Jafarnejad, S., 2019. Effect of quercetin on inflammatory factors in metabolic syndrome patients: a randomized controlled trial. *Phytotherapy Research*, 33(2), pp.262-269.

- Li, Y., Yao, J., Han, C., Yang, J., Chaudhry, M.T., Wang, S., Liu, H. and Yin, Y., 2016. Quercetin, inflammation and immunity. *Nutrients*, 8(3), p.167.

- Basil, M.C. and Levy, B.D., 2016. Specialized pro-resolving mediators: endogenous regulators of infection and inflammation. *Nature Reviews Immunology*, 16(1), pp.51-67.

- Calder, P.C., 2017. Omega-3 fatty acids and inflammatory processes: from molecules to man. *Biochemical Society Transactions*, 45(5), pp.1105-1115.

- Cutuli, D., 2017. Functional and structural benefits induced by omega-3 polyunsaturated fatty acids during aging. *Current Neuropharmacology*, 15(4), pp.534-542.

- Dyerberg, J., Madsen, P., Møller, J.M., Aardestrup, I. and Schmidt, E.B., 2010. Bioavailability of marine n-3 fatty acid formulations. *Prostaglandins, Leukotrienes and Essential Fatty Acids*, 83(3), pp.137-141.

- Kolanowski, W., Jaworska, D. and Weißbrodt, J., 2013. Importance of omega-3 long-chain polyunsaturated fatty acids in human nutrition and health. *European Food Research and Technology*, 237(5), pp.649-658.

- Serhan, C.N. and Chiang, N., 2013. Resolution phase lipid mediators of inflammation: agonists of resolution. *Current Opinion in Pharmacology*, 13(4), pp.632-640.

- Anand, P., Kunnumakkara, A.B., Newman, R.A. and Aggarwal, B.B., 2007. Bioavailability of curcumin: problems and promises. *Molecular Pharmaceutics*, 4(6), pp.807-818.

- Chandran, B. and Goel, A., 2012. A randomized, pilot study to assess the efficacy and safety of curcumin in patients with active rheumatoid arthritis. *Phytotherapy Research*, 26(11), pp.1719-1725.

- Daily, J.W., Yang, M. and Park, S., 2016. Efficacy of turmeric extracts and curcumin for alleviating the symptoms of joint arthritis: a systematic review and meta-analysis of randomized clinical trials. *Journal of Medicinal Food*, 19(8), pp.717-729.

- DiSilvestro, R.A., Joseph, E., Zhao, S. and Bomser, J., 2012. Diverse effects of a low dose supplement of lipidated curcumin in healthy middle aged people. *Nutrition Journal*, 11(1), p.79.

- Goel, A., Kunnumakkara, A.B. and Aggarwal, B.B., 2008. Curcumin as "Curecumin": from kitchen to clinic. *Biochemical Pharmacology*, 75(4), pp.787-809.

- Gupta, S.C., Patchva, S. and Aggarwal, B.B., 2013. Therapeutic roles of curcumin: lessons learned from clinical trials. *AAPS Journal*, 15(1), pp.195-218.

- Hewlings, S.J. and Kalman, D.S., 2017. Curcumin: a review of its effects on human health. *Foods*, 6(10), p.92.

- Kunnumakkara, A.B., Bordoloi, D., Padmavathi, G., Monisha, J., Roy, N.K., Prasad, S. and Aggarwal, B.B., 2017. Curcumin, the golden nutraceutical: multitargeting for multiple chronic diseases. *British Journal of Pharmacology*, 174(11), pp.1325-1348.

- Brien, S., Lewith, G., McGregor, G. and Ernst, E., 2006. Devil's Claw (Harpagophytum procumbens) as a treatment for osteoarthritis: a review of efficacy and safety. *Journal of Alternative and Complementary Medicine*, 12(10), pp.981-993.

- Chrubasik, S., Model, A., Black, A. and Pollak, S., 2003. A randomised double-blind pilot study comparing Doloteffin and Vioxx in the treatment of low back pain. *Rheumatology*, 42(5), pp.652-658.

- Chrubasik, S., Roufogalis, B.D., Wagner, H. and Chrubasik, C., 2006. A systematic review on the effectiveness of Harpagophytum extracts in the treatment of lower back pain. *Phytotherapy Research*, 20(8), pp.699-706.

- Fiebich, B.L., Muñoz, E., Rose, T., Weiss, G. and McGregor, G.P., 2012. Molecular targets of the anti-inflammatory Harpagophytum procumbens (devil's claw) extract: inhibition of TNFα and COX-2 gene expression by preventing activation of AP-1. *Phytotherapy Research*, 26(6), pp.806-811.

- Gagnier, J.J., Chrubasik, S., Manheimer, E. and Bombardier, C., 2004. Herbal medicine for low back pain: a Cochrane review. *Spine*, 29(3), pp.315-323.

- Mills, S. and Bone, K., 2013. *Principles and Practice of Phytotherapy: Modern Herbal Medicine*. 2nd ed. Edinburgh: Churchill Livingstone.

- Cani, P.D., Amar, J., Iglesias, M.A., Poggi, M., Knauf, C., Bastelica, D., Neyrinck, A.M., Fava, F., Tuohy, K.M., Chabo, C. and Waget, A., 2008. Metabolic endotoxemia initiates obesity and insulin resistance. *Diabetes*, 57(7), pp.1737-1745.

- Dai, C., Yang, J., Wen, X., Wang, D., Liu, Y. and Wu, H., 2012. *Gut*, 61(3), pp.438-449.

- Forsythe, P., Bienenstock, J. and Kunze, W.A., 2007. Vagal pathways for microbiome-brain-gut axis communication. *Advances in Experimental Medicine and Biology*, 817, pp.115-133.

- Zhang, Q., Wu, Y., Wang, J., Wu, G., Long, W., Xue, X. and Cao, Y., 2016. Probiotics and immune function: A systematic review. *Clinical Nutrition*, 35(3), pp.453-465.

Printed in Great Britain
by Amazon